Arthritis
101

Questions you have.
Answers you need.

Published by LONGSTREET PRESS, INC.,
a subsidiary of Cox Newspapers,
a division of Cox Enterprises, Inc.
2140 Newmarket Parkway
Suite 122
Marietta, Georgia 30067

Printed in the United States of America

1st printing, 1997

Library of Congress Catalog Number 96-79809

ISBN: 1-56352-380-9

Film output by OGI, Forest Park, GA

Typesetting by Jill Dible

Arthritis 101

Questions you have.
Answers you need.

TABLE OF CONTENTS

Chapter 3: Arthritis Medications — 33

Chapter 9: Diet and Arthritis — 91

Chapter 10: Joint Protection — 101

Chapter 11: Surgery — 105

Chapter 12: Unproven Remedies — 115

Chapter 13: Arthritis Research — 123

Chapter 14: Working with Arthritis: Your Legal Rights — 129

Resources — 134

Foreword

If you've just received a diagnosis of arthritis from your physician, you may very well be worried and afraid. And you may have lots and lots of questions. What does this mean? Why is this happening to me? And, most important, what happens now?

This book has the answers to many of your questions and reading it should alleviate many of your fears. For example, you'll learn that it's highly likely that your arthritis can be managed with medications and treatments, even if it is severe. Management of your arthritis will require your full participation, however. Educating yourself about your disease is a very important step toward accepting that role.

Arthritis 101 answers many basic questions about the symptoms and treatments of common types of arthritis and related conditions—osteoarthritis, rheumatoid arthritis, fibromyalgia, gout, lupus, and osteoporosis. It also provides much useful advice about how best to cope with the very real pain and discomfort arthritis causes. You will also learn about how to manage fatigue and stress, exercise and arthritis, diet and arthritis, arthritis research, and how to recognize safe and unsafe remedies. In addition, *Arthritis 101* will help you tap into the resources available in your community, through federal law and through the Arthritis Foundation, whose mission is to fund research for the cure of arthritis and improve the quality of life for people with the disease.

Arthritis affects one in every seven Americans. In part because so many people are affected, there are many sources of support and information. We encourage you to learn as much as possible about your condition so that you can take as proactive a stance as possible in its management.

Congratulations! By reading this book, you are already on your way to leading a better life with arthritis.

The Arthritis Foundation

Acknowledgments

Arthritis 101: Questions You Have. Answers You Need. is written for people who have arthritis and their family and friends. It is not meant to take the place of treatment and teaching provided by a doctor and other health-care professionals. However, it should help you understand your disease so you can take an active role in keeping it under control.

Many volunteers, physicians, health professionals and Arthritis Foundation staff contributed to *Arthritis 101: Questions You Have. Answers You Need.* Much of the book was adapted from Arthritis Foundation information booklets and *Arthritis Today* magazine. Additional information was obtained from various medical professionals.

Special thanks to the following individuals who reviewed this book: Charles R. Arkin, MD, Memphis Clinic of Internal Medicine and Rheumatology; Gerald F. Moore, MD, University of Nebraska College of Medicine; David S. Pisetsky, MD, PhD, Duke University Medical Center, Durham, NC; Terry Summerlin, MA, Memphis, TN; and Jane Zanca, Decatur, GA.

If you have any questions as you read the book, write them down and take the list with you to your doctor.

Publisher: Longstreet Press
Editorial Director: Adrienne Greer
Cover Design: Jennifer Rogers
Illustrator: Shawn Carson
Typesetter: Jill Dible
Writers: Doyt L. Conn, MD, Tracey S. Fisher, Cindy McDaniel, Krista Reese

Arthritis Foundation Reviewers:
Janet Austin, PhD, Vice President of the American Juvenile Arthritis Organization (AJAO) and Special Groups
Doyt L. Conn, MD, Senior Vice President of Medical Affairs
Leigh DeLozier, Director of Consumer Publications
Cindy McDaniel, Vice President of Publications
Susan Percy, Managing Editor, *Arthritis Today*

1

Beginning to Understand Arthritis

What exactly is arthritis?

The word *arthritis* actually refers to not just one disease but more than 100 different diseases that affect the joints as well as other parts of the body. These diseases are grouped into what are called *arthritic* or *rheumatic diseases*. Throughout this book, we will use the term *arthritis* to refer to any or all of these diseases.

The common feature in all types of arthritis is joint pain. (The literary roots of the word are the Greek words *arth*, meaning "joint," and *itis*, meaning "inflammation.") Arthritis causes pain, stiffness, and, in some cases but not all, swelling in or around the joints. Related conditions primarily affect the muscles (fibromyalgia) and the bones (osteoporosis). This book includes information to help you live better with any arthritis-related disease, as well as specific information about some common types of arthritis and related conditions, including osteoarthritis, rheumatoid arthritis, gout, and lupus.

How do I know if I have arthritis?

If you have pain, stiffness, or swelling in or around a joint that has lasted for more than two weeks, it's time to see your doctor. This is one of several

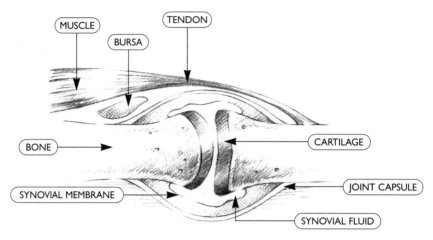

Arthritis can affect different
parts of a joint.

possible warning signs that you may have arthritis. If you are having difficulty doing everyday activities, you should be concerned. Pain from arthritis can be persistent, or it can come and go. Your joints may feel stiff or be hard to move. You may find it difficult to climb stairs, open a jar, or do other routine tasks. The pain and stiffness also may be more severe during certain times of the day, usually in the morning.

What causes arthritis?

The causes of most types of arthritis are still not known. Because there are more than 100 different types of arthritis, there may be many different causes. Scientists believe that genetics plus lifestyle and environmental factors may contribute to the development of certain types of arthritis, but the importance of these factors appears to vary with each type of arthritis.

Over the years, scientists have found that some forms of arthritis are linked to specific inherited markers (a characteristic by which a cell or molecule can be identified) called HLA proteins, which are found on the surface of cells. People with these markers appear to have a higher risk of developing certain forms of arthritis. Infections by organisms such as viruses or bacteria are another possible cause. In fact, some types of arthritis, such as Lyme disease (a bacterial infection transmitted via the bite of an infected tick), have been proven to be caused by bacteria. Research is ongoing to find out more about the causes of arthritis. (See Chapter 13 for more about this research.)

Contrary to popular belief, knuckle cracking does not cause any type of arthritis or joint degeneration. The cracking sounds that a joint makes when it is stretched, pushed, or pulled are the result of changes in pressure inside the joint capsule.

Is there a cure for arthritis?

Currently, there is no known cure for most forms of arthritis, but there are many ways to manage or control the disease, slow its course of destruction, and, if you have disability, to reduce it.

What are the components of an effective arthritis treatment plan?

Your physician can help control the symptoms of arthritis by prescribing medications that will help ease pain and slow joint damage. Physical therapy and exercise will help improve your range of motion, keep your joints flexible, and strengthen your muscles. Self-help techniques, such as relaxation exercises and participation in pain management support groups, can also help control or alleviate arthritis-related pain, fatigue, and emotional distress. Each of these treatment approaches is discussed more fully in later chapters of this book.

Should I treat myself with over-the-counter medications?

Even if you have all the symptoms discussed on page 1, it's important to visit your doctor to find out if you actually have arthritis and what type it is. The treatment your doctor will recommend will be specific to the type of arthritis you have. It's really important to know what's causing your symptoms to ensure you get fast, appropriate treatment. Getting the right treatment will make a difference in how well you do. Early diagnosis and treatment are very important to help slow or prevent joint damage, which can occur with many types of arthritis during the first few years.

Which health-care professionals treat arthritis?

A variety of health-care professionals provide medical care for people with arthritis and related conditions. Many people with arthritis are treated by *family physicians* and other primary-care physicians; these doctors' experience in diagnosing and managing arthritis-related diseases varies. *Internists* are physicians who specialize in internal medicine and in the treatment of adult diseases. They provide general treatment to adults, including adults with arthritis.

**HEALTH-CARE PROVIDERS
FOR PEOPLE WITH ARTHRITIS**

SPECIALISTS

rheumatologists, orthopaedic surgeons,
physiatrists, psychiatrists, ophthalmologists

PRIMARY CARE PHYSICIANS

family practitioners, general practitioners,
general internist, general practice
osteopaths, geriatricians
and pediatricians

ALLIED HEALTH-CARE PROFESSIONALS

physician assistants, nurse practitioners,
nurses, occupational therapists, physical
therapists, pharmacists, podiatrists,
psychologists, social workers and
vocational counselors

Among the health-care professionals who are more specifically trained to treat arthritis are *rheumatologists.* These physicians specialize in treating people with diseases that affect the joints, muscles, or bones. You may be referred to a rheumatologist to assist in your diagnosis and for recommendations concerning your treatment. (The Arthritis Foundation can provide a list of rheumatologists in your area.)

If your joints are damaged, you may be referred to an *orthopaedic surgeon* for certain surgical procedures. Other physicians who may direct part of your care include *ophthalmic specialists,* who provide eye care and treatment; *physiatrists,* who direct your physical therapy and rehabilitation; and *psychiatrists,* who treat mental or emotional problems. *Pediatricians* treat childhood diseases.

Several other professionals may also be part of your health-care team. *Occupational therapists* can teach you how to reduce strain on your joints while doing everyday activities, and *physical therapists* can show you exercises to help keep your muscles strong and your joints from becoming stiff. *Nurses, social workers* (who help find solutions to social and financial problems), *podiatrists* (foot specialists), and *psychologists* may also help with your treatment. Your physician can provide information on what professionals should be on your health-care team and who is available in your area.

What can I expect during my visit to the doctor?

There are several things you can expect to happen when you see your doctor for the first time after you suspect you have arthritis. Your doctor will ask about your medical history and your symptoms, examine you, and possibly perform some laboratory tests or X-rays.

Your doctor may move the joint that hurts or ask you to move it to assess its normal range of motion. He or she may also check for joint swelling, areas of tenderness, skin rashes, muscle weakness, or problems with other parts of your body. Your doctor may conduct laboratory tests that could include testing your blood, urine, or joint fluid. Which tests are performed will depend on what type of arthritis your doctor suspects you have developed.

The answers you give to the doctor's questions, combined with the examination and tests, will help your physician rule out other diseases that may have similar symptoms.

How can I prepare for my visit to the doctor?

You can help your doctor by writing down information about your symptoms before your visit. The more information you can provide, the better. A good place to start would be to include where you feel pain, when you experience pain, when you first began to have the pain, if you've seen any swelling or redness, and whether you've ever injured the joint. Because swelling, red-

WHAT TO TELL YOUR DOCTOR

- Where it hurts
- When it hurts
- When it first began to hurt
- How long it has hurt
- If you have seen any swelling
- What daily tasks are hard to do now
- If you have ever hurt the joint in an accident or overused it on the job or in a hobby
- If anyone in your family has had a similar problem

ness, and rashes can come and go, and because medical appointments take time to set up, it may be helpful to take photographs of your affected areas.

How does my doctor know how to treat my arthritis?

Your medical history, physical exam, and laboratory tests will help your doctor diagnose the specific type of arthritis you have and set up a treatment plan. Because there are more than 100 different types of arthritis and the pattern of joint involvement varies from one type to another, it may take more than one visit—perhaps even several visits—for your doctor to determine just what type of arthritis you have. The symptoms of some types of arthritis develop slowly and may appear similar to the symptoms that occur in the early stages of other diseases.

How important is getting a second opinion about my diagnosis and treatment?

If at some point you're not satisfied with your diagnosis or treatment, it's all right to seek an opinion from another doctor. For the name of a qualified rheumatologist, call your local Arthritis Foundation chapter, the American College of Rheumatology, or a local university arthritis center. Ask that a copy of your medical records be sent to the consulting physician. The consulting physician will usually call or write your physician stating his or her findings and providing advice for treatment. Discuss the second opinion with your own doctor. A good doctor's feelings should not be hurt because you are seeking a second opinion. In fact, your doctor may thank you for helping to improve your care.

What is a flare?

People with some types of rheumatic diseases, such as rheumatoid arthritis or lupus, experience periods when their disease becomes worse and periods when it improves. A *flare* is the term used to describe the times when the disease is at its worst. If you have one of the types of arthritis that causes flares, you may have more stiffness, pain, swelling, and fatigue during flares than usual.

What is remission?

Remission is the term used to describe the period of time when the symptoms of a disease improve or even disappear completely. No one can predict when or if symptoms will cease, or how long remission will last. Remission is often medication-induced, which illustrates how well some types of arthritis can be managed with medication. If you think your disease is in remission, it is important not to stop your medication without consulting your physician.

Will living in a warmer climate improve my arthritis?

Some people with arthritis feel better in a warm, dry climate. For people with arthritis, life can be easier in a warm climate, because they don't have to struggle with ice and snow. Studies of the effects of weather on people with rheumatoid arthritis are inconclusive. Symptoms may worsen if the barometric pressure goes down and the humidity goes up. And even if the warmer, drier climate helps you feel better, it will not alleviate the disease itself. If you are considering a move to a warmer climate, spending more than a vacation there will be necessary to assess how your symptoms are affected. Another thing to consider before moving is the effect of moving away from your support system of family and friends, which may outweigh the benefits of the warmer weather.

Can I get health-care coverage if I have arthritis?

In most cases, you can get health insurance if you have arthritis, but it may not be as easy for you as it is for others. That's because most rheumatic conditions are chronic, meaning they may last a lifetime, and many health plans are concerned that it will cost too much to care for you. You may also have needs that other people don't have—visits to specialists, medications, physical or occupational therapy, and assistive devices. There should be a plan that fits your needs, and choosing the right plan is important.

How do I obtain coverage with a pre-existing condition?

If you have arthritis, you may be classified as a higher risk to insure because you have what insurance companies call a pre-existing condition. This is an illness or injury for which you have received treatment, or for which a reasonable prudent person should have sought treatment during a specified time (usually six months to a year), before the insurance policy was issued.

When considering a health-care plan, pay particular attention to clauses that indicate the insurer denies coverage to people with chronic diseases, including arthritis. In the past, some plans offered coverage for care related to a pre-existing illness but required the insured to pay excessive premiums, deductibles, or co-payments; some plans imposed a waiting period of longer than one year; and some plans limited services for a person's condition in number, type, and dollar amount because it is a pre-existing condition.

However, the new Health Insurance Reform Act, signed into law as P.L. 104-191 on August 21, 1996, will protect persons who already have health coverage from losing it. The law guarantees that individuals who lose or leave their jobs can maintain health insurance coverage, even if they are sick.

CHECKLIST FOR CHOOSING A HEALTH PLAN

TO FIND THE POLICY THAT BEST MEETS YOUR NEEDS, GET ANSWERS TO THE FOLLOWING QUESTIONS:

- **Cost:** What is the average annual cost of coverage, including premiums, deductibles and co-payments?

- **Limitations:** Is there a waiting period or are there coverage limitations for pre-existing conditions?

- **Drugs:** If the plan has a prescription drug benefit, can the most effective arthritis drugs be prescribed without financial disincentives to the physician or patient?

- **Coverage:** Does the plan provide coverage for prescribed therapy and/or orthotics? Are there limits on where you may go for therapy?

- **Choice:** Are there limits on your choice of doctors or health-care facilities? Can you request referrals to a subspecialist?

- **Limits:** Are there limitations on where you can have labwork drawn or X-rays taken?

- **Approval:** Do diagnostic tests require prior approval?

- **Board certification:** Does the health plan include a board-eligible or board-certified rheumatologist?

- **Specially-trained surgeons:** Are there orthopaedic surgeons who have special skills in arthritis-related problems?

- **Payment:** How is the physician paid? Does the physician take a financial risk in determining your treatment plan or by providing your care?

The law will limit to twelve months the period in which a group insurer could refuse or limit coverage of a new enrollee for a health condition that was treated or diagnosed in the six-month period before enrollment. The twelve month period would be reduced by the period of continuous coverage before enrollment.

Compliance for most of these provisions will begin July 1, 1997, and enforcement will begin January 1, 1998.

Even with a pre-existing condition, you can still get coverage through a managed care plan, especially if you join through a group plan. In this case, you may have a waiting period before being covered for your pre-existing condition, but you will still have coverage for new health problems that may arise after your coverage begins. The plan should also cover your pre-existing condition after the exclusion period has elapsed. Each plan has different clauses having to do with pre-existing conditions, so examine them carefully.

Pre-existing condition clauses can be confusing. It's important to read your policy carefully so that you know what will be covered and what won't.

What are the other limitations in coverage if I have arthritis?

Insurance carriers have traditionally limited their financial risk by limiting how much they will pay for rehabilitation services, durable medical equipment, and arthritis medications. As a result, some people with arthritis have been denied sufficient coverage or have been forced to seek services from the public-health sector or to go without needed treatments. Managed care is intended as a sensible alternative to these arbitrary limitations. Managed care organizations have increasingly developed techniques that allow coverage for appropriate medication and services while still controlling costs. These techniques include methods for managing clients' access to services and treatment as well as methods for paying health-care providers.

How do I find the right health plan?

Many organizations can give you information about health-care plans in your area that will make it easier to choose wisely. Call your local Arthritis Foundation or contact any of the following sources:

- *Employers:* Health benefits managers can give you valuable information about choosing a health-care plan. Ask for charts, pamphlets, and survey results, as well as statistics showing complaints to the employer about these plans.

• *Health-care providers:* Many health-care providers who treat people with arthritis belong to provider networks. If your provider is a member of a managed care organization, ask for a list of the plans with which he or she is affiliated. Determine whether your employer offers these plans or whether you can join in another manner. Usually these plans must be selected during an open enrollment period. Before selecting a plan, compare plan premiums, benefits, indicators of quality, and other data.

Ask your physician for recommendations of which plan to join. You can also ask your physician what other patients have said about particular plans. The Arthritis Foundation has a booklet that may help you choose a health plan. Call 800/207-8633 to order a copy of *Choosing A Health Plan.*

2

Common Arthritis-Related Diseases and Conditions

This chapter offers a brief introduction to six common arthritis-related diseases and conditions: osteoarthritis, rheumatoid arthritis, fibromyalgia, gout, lupus, and osteoporosis, plus a quick look at juvenile rheumatoid arthritis. You'll learn about the symptoms and causes of each of these conditions as well as treatment options.

There are many other types of arthritis-related conditions, including ankylosing spondylitis, back pain, bursitis and tendinitis, carpal tunnel syndrome, Lyme disease, scleroderma, and Sjögren's syndrome, to name a few. Because there are more than 100 kinds of arthritis, it's important to know which type you have to treat it properly. Although each type isn't specifically discussed in this chapter, the information and advice throughout this book are applicable to most arthritis-related conditions.

What is osteoarthritis?

Osteoarthritis (OA), also called degenerative arthritis, is a disease that results from the breakdown of cartilage in joints, leading to joint pain and damage. Almost 16 million people in the United States have osteoarthritis, making it one of the most common diseases.

The joints most commonly affected by osteoarthritis are the end joints of the fingers, the base of the thumb, and the hip, knee, and the joints of the lower back. Usually the affected joint or joints hurt most after overuse or after periods of inactivity, and there may be some stiffness in the mornings.

If you have osteoarthritis and don't move and exercise the sore joint, the muscles surrounding the joint may become weaker and sometimes smaller in size. As a result, the weak muscles won't be able to support the joint as well and you may have increased pain with use. If the hip or knee is involved, you may also notice that your coordination and posture are not as good as they were before you had osteoarthritis.

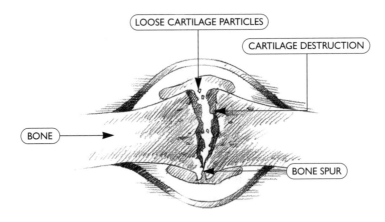

Joint with osteoarthritis

What causes osteoarthritis?

Several factors increase the risk of developing osteoarthritis. Older people are more likely to develop the disease, and women develop the disease in larger numbers than men. Other risk factors include genetic predisposition, obesity, repetitive biomechanical stresses on a particular joint or joints, trauma, and congenital abnormalities, such as being born with a knock-knee deformity.

How is osteoarthritis diagnosed?

As with all types of arthritis, a doctor usually diagnoses OA based on a medical history and a physical examination. The doctor may also require some other procedures and/or tests, such as X-rays, to help confirm the diagnosis, to determine how much joint damage has occurred, and to help rule out other kinds of arthritis.

By talking with you, your physician will learn which joint or joints are bothering you. Then, by examining you, he or she will see if the joint is swollen or enlarged and if that joint is functioning normally or has a limited range of motion. By determining joint abnormalities, knowing that osteoarthritis affects certain joints in a particular manner, and obtaining X-rays of the joint and observing cartilage loss and possibly bony overgrowth, your doctor will be able to determine if you have osteoarthritis.

How is osteoarthritis treated?

If you have osteoarthritis, the goals of your treatment program will be to control your pain, minimize functional limitations and associated disability, and, of course, balance the risks of any drug use with potential benefits. The first component of osteoarthritis management will be to help you understand the disease and what you can do to help yourself.

If you have osteoarthritis of a knee or hip and are overweight, it is important to get involved in a weight reduction program. It will also be important to strengthen the muscles surrounding the joint. This can be done with the guidance and help of a physical therapist. If there is significant impairment of joint function and you are having difficulty walking any distance, then your physical therapist may suggest an assistive device, such as a cane, to take the weight off the involved joint when walking. If the finger joints are involved, the physical therapist and an occupational therapist will help you modify the way you use your hands so as to minimize the harmful effects of certain activities. The occupational therapist may also recommend certain splints.

In addition to maintaining range of motion of the involved joint and strengthening muscles surrounding the joint, your physical therapist will also want you to be involved in some type of conditioning program. This will depend on which joint or joints are involved, what physical activities you like, and what activities are available. Your exercise program will be tailored to you.

What about drugs to help manage osteoarthritis?

The principal role of drug treatment in osteoarthritis is to control pain. There are no drugs available that have been shown to reverse the cartilage damage associated with osteoarthritis or to prevent the progression of joint abnormalities. Consequently, your physician will recommend medications that help control pain but that do not put you at great risk for side effects. Acetaminophen is frequently used to help control the pain of osteoarthritis because it is relatively safe.

If there is inflammation of the joint, there will be additional swelling and sometimes warmth around the joint. By removing and analyzing the fluid from the joint, your physician will be able to determine if there is inflammation. If there is, he or she may want you to take a nonsteroidal anti-inflammatory drug (NSAID). NSAIDs are associated with an increased risk of irritating the stomach and in older people can be associated with other side effects; however, all medicines, including acetaminophen, have side effects, and, after considering the pros and cons, your physician may still recommend an NSAID. (For further information, see page 33 on NSAIDs and page 35 on side effects.)

What other treatment options may be available?

If one joint is persistently painful and swollen, your physician may want to aspirate the joint; this involves removing some joint fluid so it can be analyzed for the presence of crystals and to determine the amount of inflammation you have. At the same time, your physician may inject corticosteroids into the joint to help control the pain and inflammation. If you have a joint that is persistently painful and has severely limited your ability to function, such as severe involvement of the knee or hip, your physician may refer you to an orthopaedic surgeon to determine if joint surgery is the best course of action. Joint-replacement surgery for the hips and knees is very effective in controlling the pain in those joints and improving function.

What is the best way to manage osteoarthritis?

The best way to manage your osteoarthritis is by learning as much as you can about the disease and how it affects you. This will require that you work with your physician. You can prepare for your visit to your physician by writing down your observations about how your joint or joints are affected by your osteoarthritis and how your activities are limited. Talk with your family and friends to get their perspectives and share information with them.

Remember, you can play an important role in helping yourself manage your disease. If you are overweight, you can help yourself—and your joints—by getting your weight down to a reasonable level. You can work with your physician in strengthening the muscles around the joint and conditioning your body. The earlier the problem is recognized and you get started on a good management program, the better you will do.

What is an autoimmune disease?

The immune system is your body's natural defense against antigens, which are substances your body regards as foreign. Bacteria and viruses are examples of antigens. The immune system fights off antigens by producing antibodies, whose job it is to render the antigens harmless.

Occasionally, the immune system does not function properly and loses the ability to distinguish between its own body cells and antigens, causing the antibodies to mistakenly fight the body's own cells. This is referred to as an autoimmune response (*auto* means "self"). The damage that occurs from an autoimmune response may take the form of inflammation and injury to body tissues and organs. Rheumatoid arthritis and lupus are two arthritis-related autoimmune diseases in which this damage affects the joints as well as other parts of the body.

What is rheumatoid arthritis?

Rheumatoid arthritis (RA) is a common form of arthritis that can lead to deformity. It is the result of inflammation of the lining of joints and sometimes joint tissues. Joint inflammation is characterized by pain, swelling, limitation of motion, and sometimes redness over the joint. The inflammation associated with RA may also affect other parts of the body, such as the eyes, skin, peripheral nerves that supply the extremities (arms and legs), and the lining of the tissues around the heart and lungs.

Certain joints are commonly involved in RA, including the small joints of the hands and feet, wrists, elbows, shoulders, jaws, neck; and the ankles, hips, and knees. The potential for joint damage and the frequent presence of *rheumatoid factor* (an antibody in the blood) distinguish RA from other types of arthritis such as osteoarthritis.

Rheumatoid arthritis may follow a variety of courses. The disease may occur slowly and involve only one joint and then progress to involve other joints. Or it may come on suddenly and involve many joints all at once. RA may be accompanied by pain and stiffness in many joints plus fever, weight loss, fatigue, and an elevated erythrocyte sedimentation rate (ESR), which your doctor can detect with a blood test. (See "How Is RA Diagnosed?")

Adults with rheumatoid arthritis may have rheumatoid nodules, inflamed knots or bumps that appear over pressure areas such as the elbow. Sometimes patients with more severe disease experience inflammation of the peripheral nerves that supply the extremities (arms and legs), resulting in numbness, tingling, pain, and sometimes weakness of the muscles supplied by those nerves. Skin inflammation may also be present, resulting in sores and ulcers of the lower legs.

What causes RA?

Although the exact cause of RA is not known, researchers have established that genetics (or heredity) play at least some role in the development of the disease. (See page 124 for information on research on RA.) Evidence of genetic associations have been found in several racial populations, but the association is not the same in each racial group. Even if an exact genetic link could be found, however, it is unlikely that genetics alone bring about the disease.

Researchers suspect that one or more infectious agents may trigger the initial inflammation of the joint lining that leads to a diagnosis of rheumatoid arthritis in susceptible people. Once that trigger occurs, inflammatory cells stay "turned on," causing the inflammation to continue.

How is RA diagnosed?

A physician who is knowledgeable and experienced in dealing with RA can diagnose the disease based on a medical history, physical examination and selected laboratory tests.

The first step in diagnosis is to recognize that something is wrong, that you are not feeling well, and that one or more joints are painful and don't function right. If this is the case, you should go to your physician and explain your problems. Your physician will take your medical history and examine you. The pattern of your joint involvement will help your doctor determine the type of arthritis you have. If your physician detects swelling in a number of joints as well as rheumatoid nodules over your elbows or in other pressure areas, you likely have RA.

To confirm the diagnosis, your physician may order certain laboratory tests and X-rays of selected joints. If you have RA, you may have an antibody in your blood called rheumatoid factor. Your doctor may perform a test that

OSTEOARTHRITIS	RHEUMATOID ARTHRITIS
Usually begins after age 40	Usually begins between ages of 25 and 50
Usually develops slowly over many years	May develop suddenly within weeks or months
Often affects joints on only one side of the body at first	Usually affects joints on both sides of the body (e.g., both knees)
Usually doesn't cause redness, warmth or swelling of joints	Causes redness, warmth and swelling of joints
Affects only certain joints; rarely affects elbows, shoulders or ankles	Affects many joints, usually small joints of the hands and feet, and may include elbows, shoulders or ankles
Doesn't cause a general feeling of sickness	Often causes a general feeling of sickness and fatigue, as well as weight loss and fever

detects and measures the level of this antibody.

Another test that your doctor may order determines your erythrocyte sedimentation rate (ESR or sed rate), which may be elevated. This test measures how fast red blood cells cling together, fall, and settle (like sediment) in the bottom of a glass tube over the course of an hour. The higher the rate, the greater the amount of inflammation.

Your doctor may also test to see if your red blood cell count is depressed, indicating that you have anemia. Anemia is a common condition in which fewer than normal red blood cells are present. Your doctor may also order a *platelet count*, to measure the number of cells in the blood that help it to clot.

Although these blood tests can be helpful in making a diagnosis, there is no single blood test that can establish or exclude the diagnosis of RA. Early in the course of RA there may be no abnormalities detected in the blood or on joint X-rays.

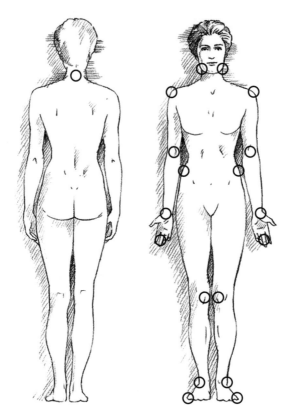

Joints that may be affected by RA

How is RA treated?

Although there is not yet a cure for RA, the disease can be managed well with medications and other treatments. The earlier the diagnosis is made and treatment instituted, the greater the chance that the disease can be controlled with minimal joint damage. If you have been diagnosed with RA, your physician will likely treat you with an NSAID. He or she may also start you on a disease-modifying drug, such as methotrexate or hydroxychloroquine. If you are experiencing a lot of pain and stiffness in many joints, your physician may also add low doses of a cortisone-type medicine called Prednisone. (See Chapter 3 for more information on medications for RA.)

If you have RA, it is important to be followed regularly by a physician experienced in its management who can detect any problems with medications and adjust medications to allow the best control of your condition. With the information and medications available today, it should be possible to manage your arthritis quite well.

What other treatments are effective in managing RA?

Your physician will help you understand your disease and the recommended medications so that you know why you are taking them and what to expect.

Your physician will likely send you to a physical therapist and an occupational therapist to show you how to protect your joints, function better, and maintain good range of motion. When the active inflammation is controlled, your physician and physical therapist will help you strengthen the muscles around the joints and eventually will recommend an exercise program tailored for you.

Other strategies are available to help you improve and deal with your disease. The Arthritis Foundation sponsors support groups, exercise programs, and disease management programs, such as the *Arthritis Self-Help Course*. These strategies are important in helping you understand your disease and equally important in helping you cope with it.

Even if you have already developed damage in a number of joints, there is still much you can do to manage the disease. Most of the medications and strategies described above will still be effective. Your physician may have an occupational therapist develop splints for joints that are heavily affected by the arthritis. If you have significant destruction of a joint, resulting in chronic pain and disability, your doctor may refer you to an orthopaedic surgeon to discuss joint-replacement surgery.

Whether the RA is in the early stages of development and mild or it has been present for years, resulting in joint destruction, there are ways to live better with it. It is important that you work with your physician and take your medications as prescribed, even if you are feeling better.

You and your family should learn all you can about the disease and talk about it with each other, with your doctors, and with the other professionals on your health-care team. Using medications properly, developing good health practices, getting appropriate amounts of rest and exercise, and learning how to cope with emotional stress are all proactive steps you can take to help yourself control the illness.

What is lupus?

Systemic lupus erythematosus (also called SLE or lupus) is an inflammatory disease that can affect various internal organs. Although the disease has a variable course and outcome, the prognosis has improved significantly over the last decade. Lupus is more common in women, particularly during their childbearing years, and among the African-American population.

What causes lupus?

Although the exact cause of lupus is not known, doctors and scientists agree that it is an autoimmune disease. In addition, the effect of age and sex on the occurrence of lupus suggests that hormonal factors play a role in the development of the disease. There is a high prevalence of lupus among identical twins, and a relatively high percentage (approximately 10 percent) of first-degree (immediate) relatives of people with lupus develop the disease, indicating that genetic factors may also play a role.

What are the symptoms of lupus?

Although the symptoms and features of lupus vary, three of the most common symptoms are fever, a rash, and arthritis. The skin rash may be triggered by sun exposure and may occur in areas of the skin that have been exposed to the sun. It may take the form of a butterfly-shaped rash over the cheeks and across the bridge of the nose (known as a malar rash), or there may be diffuse redness, hives, painful red spots, hair loss, or sores.

Other symptoms of lupus may include fatigue, weight loss, and generalized stiffness with pain and swelling in several joints. There may also be inflammation of the lining around the heart, lungs, or abdomen, causing pain when you take a deep breath.

Other potentially serious features of lupus may include inflammation of the kidneys, causing protein in the urine, reduced kidney function, and high blood pressure; inflammation within the brain, which can cause seizures; or inflammation in the bone marrow, which can cause anemia and a reduction in the numbers of white blood cells and platelets.

How is lupus diagnosed?

Lupus may be difficult to diagnose initially because the symptoms and signs vary and may resemble those of other diseases. For that reason, it is important to see a doctor who is knowledgeable and experienced in treating rheumatic diseases.

In addition to the features described above, people with lupus usually have what are known as antinuclear antibodies in their blood. If your physician suspects you have lupus, he or she may order a blood test to detect these antinuclear antibodies, as well as a blood count, a urinalysis, and kidney function tests. These tests will determine the extent of inflammation in your system and which organs are involved.

How is lupus treated?

How lupus is treated depends on which organs are involved, the activity of the disease, and the extent of disease. Joint pain and stiffness may be managed with an NSAID. If there is inflammation of the skin, depending on its severity, your physician may prescribe steroid creams or low doses of prednison to be taken orally. If the disease is affecting the lining of the heart and lungs, a kidney, or the central nervous system, or, if there is a lowering of your platelet count, higher doses of Prednisone may be required. Usually, hydroxychloroquine (*Plaquenil*) is used in addition to an NSAID and the low doses of Prednisone to aid in the long-term management of joint, skin, and organ involvement. If there is more serious involvement of a kidney or the central nervous system, a cytotoxic agent, such as cyclophosphamide (*Cytoxan*) or azathioprine (*Imuran*), may be used in addition to Prednisone for control of these inflammatory manifestations. (See Chapter 3 for more on arthritis medications.)

If you have lupus, it is important that you take good care of yourself. You should adhere to a diet low in salt and fats, and you should exercise regularly. Which forms of exercise will be best for you may depend on which organs or joints are involved and the extent to which they are diseased. Smoking is harmful for everyone but particularly if you have lupus, because nicotine exacerbates the inflammation of the small blood vessels affected by lupus. Controlling high blood pressure is also important.

Social and emotional support is essential for anyone living with a chronic disease such as lupus. Support groups are available through the Arthritis Foundation and the Lupus Foundation. They can be very important in achieving emotional health and maintaining a positive attitude. It is important to remember, though, that you may not experience some of the problems that others with lupus do. Reading the latest information about lupus is another way to learn more about how it affects your body and how to deal with it.

What exactly is gout?

Gout is a rheumatic disease that causes sudden, severe episodes of pain and tenderness, redness, warmth, and swelling (inflammation) in some joints. Gout results when the body makes too much or is unable to get rid of a naturally-occurring substance in the body called *uric acid*.

Uric acid is a chemical that normally is formed when the body breaks down substances called purines found inside cells. Sometimes eating too much meat and consuming too much alcohol will increase the levels of uric acid. Hereditary factors may also be important.

Uric acid is ordinarily dissolved in the blood and passed through the kidneys into the urine. In people with gout, the uric acid level in the blood is high and may be deposited in the joint tissue. There, the uric acid may form needle-like crystals in the joint that trigger inflammation and cause pain and swelling.

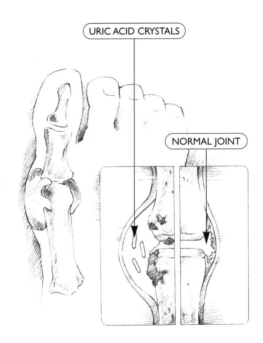

Joint with gout

FOODS THAT MAY RAISE URIC ACID LEVELS

If you have gout, you may need to completely avoid these foods: sardines, anchovies, brain, kidney, liver, sweetbreads and other animal meats.

What are the symptoms of gout?

Gout usually affects one joint at a time; initially, this is often the large joint of the big toe. It can also affect other joints, such as the knee, ankle, foot, hand, wrist, and elbow. It may start in one joint and later involve other joints.

Attacks of gout frequently occur after unaccustomed stress, such as walking too much or consuming too much alcohol, or after a serious illness or accident. During an episode, people with gout may experience sudden and severe joint pain, joint swelling, shiny red or purple skin around the joint, and extreme tenderness in the joint area. The attack may last a number of days.

Who gets gout?

Gout affects more than one million Americans from all walks of life. It most often affects men between the ages of 40 and 50 who have a family history of gout, are overweight, hypertensive, and consume too much alcohol. It also affects postmenopausal women, particularly those on diuretics (medications that increase the amount of urine excreted) and who are overweight. Gout may be difficult to diagnose because it may occur on top of a joint damaged by osteoarthritis, and the diagnosis of gout may not be considered.

How is gout diagnosed?

Before your doctor will be able to diagnose you with gout, he or she will ask you to describe your symptoms and will examine you. Your doctor may measure the amount of uric acid in your blood and may also want to rule out other types of arthritis that resemble gout. He or she will most likely need to remove fluid from an affected joint and examine it for the presence of crystals. This is the best way to diagnose gout.

How is gout treated?

The treatment of gout consists of taking medications to control the inflammation and to reduce the level of uric acid in the blood. If you have been diagnosed with gout, your doctor will treat your initial attack with a potent nonsteroidal anti-inflammatory drug or with colchicine, a medication that controls inflammation. Anti-inflammatory medications control the inflammation, pain, swelling, and redness caused by the formation of uric acid crystals in the joint.

If you have experienced repeated attacks, or if there is evidence of uric acid deposits under the skin (known as tophi) then your doctor will probably want to use medications to reduce the uric acid level in the blood or to increase the excretion of uric acid in the kidneys. The drug that reduces the production of uric acid is called allopurinol *(Lopurin, Zyloprim),* and the drug that increases the excretion of uric acid through the kidneys is called probenicid *(Benemid).* Your doctor will decide which one is best for you. If your doctor prescribes one of these drugs, he or she will also prescribe either an NSAID or colchicine in low doses for several months to reduce the likelihood of your having an attack of gout during the process of lowering the uric acid level in your blood.

Is there a cure for gout?

Acute gout attacks can be cured with medication and future attacks prevented if the diagnosis is made early and appropriate treatment instituted. Adhering to the treatment plan as well as the diet prescribed by the doctor are equally important.

What is fibromyalgia?

Fibromyalgia is a form of soft-tissue rheumatism (a condition marked by stiffness and pain in the muscles and tissues around the joints), rather than arthritis of a joint. The term "fibromyalgia" means pain in the muscles and the fibrous connective tissues (the *ligaments* and *tendons*). Fibromyalgia is characterized by persistent pain in the muscles and soft tissues. People with fibromyalgia may feel as though they have a joint disease, but fibromyalgia is not a true form of arthritis and does not cause joint damage.

Fibromyalgia is often misunderstood because there are no joint abnormalities, weaknesses, or limitations of function. The person, at least on the outside, appears to be perfectly fine.

What are the symptoms of fibromyalgia?

Pain and fatigue are the most prominent symptoms of fibromyalgia. The pain is typically felt all over, although it may start in one region, such as the neck and shoulders. There are usually sensitive areas known as tender points or trigger points in certain parts of the body that aid physicians in their diagnosis.

Fibromyalgia pain has been described as burning, sore, and aching. The time of the day, activity level, weather, sleep patterns, and stress can all contribute to its severity. Many people with fibromyalgia say that they are always in pain to some degree. About 90 percent of people with fibromyalgia describe feeling moderate to severe fatigue coupled with a lack of energy, decreased endurance during exercise, or even the kind of exhaustion you feel when you have the flu or are suffering from lack of sleep.

People with fibromyalgia may also feel anxious, depressed, or angry. These feelings may get worse the longer the pain lasts and, in turn, may magnify the pain.

What causes fibromyalgia?

Many factors are suspected to trigger this disorder. A prior illness, physical or emotional trauma, chronic stress, depression, inactivity, or overuse of muscles may contribute to the fatigue, poor sleep patterns, and resulting vicious cycle of pain that characterize fibromyalgia. Because people with fibromyalgia are in pain, they may not experience restorative sleep: Their muscles do not relax while they're sleeping, which results in further pain and fatigue.

Investigators are studying the possibility that abnormalities in certain body chemicals, including serotonin and substance P, might be associated with and in some way contribute to the symptoms of fibromyalgia. Likewise, scientists are studying brain function and brain blood flow in fibromyalgia patients.

How is fibromyalgia treated?

Treatment of fibromyalgia currently includes medication to diminish the pain and provide more restorative sleep, exercises to strengthen muscles and improve cardiovascular fitness, relaxation techniques to ease tense muscles, and educational programs to develop coping skills. As with most chronic conditions, treatment should be tailored to meet individual needs.

If you have fibromyalgia, your physician may prescribe several medications to help minimize your symptoms. Antidepressants help promote deeper sleep and often reduce pain. Anti-inflammatory medications used to treat arthritis do not have a major benefit in patients with fibromyalgia, but modest doses of over-the-counter anti-inflammatory medications, such as aspirin and ibuprofen, may provide some pain relief. Analgesics such as acetaminophen may also provide some relief. Narcotic pain relievers, tranquilizers, and cortisone derivatives (steroids) are not effective and should be avoided because of their potential side effects. (See Chapter 3 for more on medications.)

If you have fibromyalgia, your own active involvement in the management of your condition is a key component of treatment. Learn as much as possible about your condition. In the process, you will learn that you hold the key to your improvement. By taking charge, developing a positive attitude, getting involved in a tailored exercise program, and working with knowledgeable and empathetic professionals, you will improve.

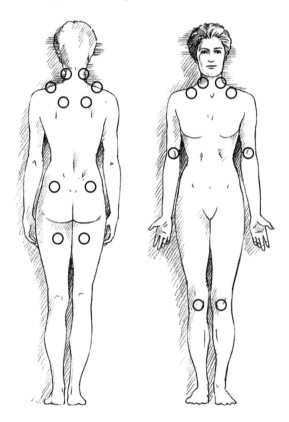

Tender points are
common in fibromyalgia.

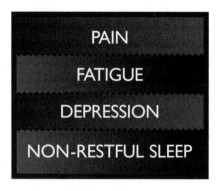

PAIN

FATIGUE

DEPRESSION

NON-RESTFUL SLEEP

These factors may contribute
to fibromyalgia symptoms.

What's the prognosis for people with fibromyalgia?

In the search for the cause of their discomfort and pain, people with fibromyalgia often undergo many tests and see many specialists. Sometimes people with fibromyalgia are told that since they look well, they aren't suffering from a real disorder and are dismissed. Fear and frustration often result, which in turn may increase the pain.

If you have fibromyalgia, it is important to remember that it is not life-threatening and causes no visible changes in the body. Although symptoms may vary, the condition will not deform or cripple. For many people, just knowing that fibromyalgia is not a deforming disease allows them to discontinue expensive testing and develop a more positive attitude about their condition.

At the same time, fibromyalgia should be taken seriously and dealt with as you would any problem that causes chronic pain and fatigue. It is important to recognize that the pain and suffering of fibromyalgia is real and can be frustrating and debilitating. However, with the help of a knowledgeable physician and other members of your health-care team with whom you feel comfortable, your condition can be managed and improved.

The Arthritis Foundation has a self-help workbook to help people with fibromyalgia better manage their condition. Visit your local bookstore or call 800/207-8633 to order *Your Personal Guide to Living Better with Fibromyalgia.*

What is osteoporosis?

Osteoporosis is a disease that causes bones to lose their mass and break easily. The word *osteoporosis* means "bone that is porous." Osteoporosis is a serious public health problem in the United States, affecting more than 24 million people and causing more than 1.5 million fractures each year. It is the major underlying cause of bone fractures in postmenopausal women and the elderly. Osteoporosis is a completely different disease from osteoarthritis, described earlier in this chapter.

Who gets osteoporosis?

Women are more likely to get osteoporosis than men, and postmenopausal Caucasian and Asian women with small, thin frames are at greatest risk. The incidence of hip fractures goes up rapidly after the age of 50 in women and after the age of 60 in men.

There are several reasons women are at increased risk of developing osteoporosis. First, their bones are 20 to 30 percent less dense than those of men; consequently, women have less bone to lose. Second, estrogen is important in maintaining women's bones, but after menopause, women's estrogen levels drop dramatically, which contributes to accelerated bone loss.

Too little calcium and vitamin D in the diet, as well as too little exercise, can increase a person's risk of developing osteoporosis. A lack of exercise can also reduce a person's agility, which, in turn, increases the likelihood of a fall. The use of sedatives, diuretic drugs and alcohol may also increase the risk of falls, especially in the elderly. High-heeled shoes, as well as slippery floors, small area rugs, and bathrooms without guardrails, may also be hazardous.

Women with inflammatory diseases, such as rheumatoid arthritis and lupus, are at even greater risk of developing osteoporosis because the inflammation caused by these diseases and the use of corticosteroids (Prednisone), frequently prescribed to treat these diseases, both cause and accelerate the development of osteoporosis.

What happens to the bones when someone has osteoporosis?

Throughout life, your bone undergoes a process called remodeling, in which old bone is broken down and replaced with strong new bone. Until approximately age 30, the rate at which bone is replaced is greater than the rate at which it is broken down. By the time you reach your early 30s, your bone mass is generally at its peak—your bones are as dense and as strong as they'll ever be.

Sometime after this point, bone mass levels off, and eventually the rate at which bone breaks down becomes greater than the rate at which it can be replaced. This bone loss is accelerated in women after menopause because of the drop in their estrogen levels. If the breakdown occurs too rapidly or the replacement too slowly, the bone becomes more porous and, thus, weaker.

How will I know if I have osteoporosis?

Bones with less mass are more likely to break or fracture, even in a minor fall. The first warning or symptom of osteoporosis may be a broken bone. In other instances, silent fractures of the spine result in both a loss of height and rounded shoulders, often referred to as a dowager's hump.

Even before these symptoms appear, there are tests that can determine if you have osteoporosis. Your doctor may ask you questions about symptoms, especially when and where you feel pain. He or she may ask you about your medical history, including your overall health, previous illnesses, past fractures, diet, and medications. A physical examination and blood and urine tests may be done to rule out other diseases that weaken bone.

Although information from your medical history and physical examination can be helpful, the only sure way to determine the density of your bones is through a bone density measurement test. Instruments to measure bone density include CT (computed tomography) and DEXA (dual-energy X-ray absorptiometry) scans. Regular bone X-rays may show fractures, but only bone density measurement tests will show significant reduced density.

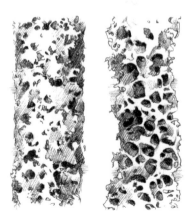

Osteoporosis makes bones less dense,
as is evident in the bone on the right.

WHAT ARE THE RISK FACTORS?

YOU MAY BE MORE SUSCEPTIBLE TO OSTEOPOROSIS IF YOU:

- are of Caucasian or Asian ancestry;
- have a low intake of calcium-rich foods, such as dairy foods;
- consume or take insufficient amounts of vitamin D;
- are menopausal or have had ovaries removed;
- are thin and have a small frame;
- have low levels of testosterone (men only);
- use medications that reduce bone mass (cortisone, anticonvulsants or heparin);
- smoke;
- drink more than two alcoholic beverages a day; and/or
- do not exercise regularly.

If you have several of these risk factors, you are at greater risk of breaking a bone and should talk to your doctor about it during your next appointment.

How is osteoporosis treated?

One of the most effective "treatments" for osteoporosis is prevention in people with identified risk factors. This prevention may take the form of estrogen replacement therapy in postmenopausal women, or nutrition or exercise counseling.

Once osteoporosis develops, the treatment may depend on the symptoms. If the first recognition of osteoporosis is with the first fracture, the physician must manage that fracture and associated pain. The management will depend on where the fracture is located. If it is a compression fracture of the spine, your doctor will prescribe bed rest. If it is a wrist fracture, the management will include the use of a cast. If it is a hip fracture, surgery may be needed to repair or replace the hip. In all of these situations, your doctor will manage the pain with appropriate medications, which may include narcotics for a while.

After the fracture and pain have been managed, treatment will focus on preventing any worsening of the osteoporosis. Your physician will want you to take sufficient amounts of calcium and vitamin D. If you are not taking estrogen, and there is no reason not to take it, your physician may prescribe estrogen and possibly a progestational agent as well. At the same time, your physician will get you started on an exercise program that will be tailored to you and your particular problem. It will be important to keep your muscles strong and to improve your coordination and balance.

Your physician may also consider using other drugs to slow down the bone loss caused by the osteoporosis. These drugs include alendrenate (*Fosamax*) and calcitonin (*Calcimar*, *Miacalcin*). The use of these medications will depend on whether or not you are on estrogen or can take estrogen and on the severity of your osteoporosis. Your physician will know when to consider these other medications.

Does arthritis affect children?

About 200,000 children in the United States have some form of arthritis. The most common form in children is juvenile rheumatoid arthritis (JRA). However, children may also be affected by arthritis as a feature of other diseases, including lupus (see page 20); juvenile dermatomyositis (a disease that causes a skin rash and weak muscles in children and that may be accompanied by swollen joints); and the spondylarthropathies of childhood (diseases that involve the joints and later the spine), to name a few.

What is juvenile rheumatoid arthritis?

Juvenile rheumatoid arthritis (JRA) affects about 70,000 children in the United States. It is a disease of the joints that may also affect other organs. JRA is often a mild condition that causes few problems, but in severe cases it can produce serious complications. Its signs and symptoms may change frequently. Joint stiffness and pain may be mild one day but become so severe the next that the child cannot move without great difficulty.

There are at least three forms of juvenile rheumatoid arthritis. Each form begins in a different way and has different signs and symptoms. These three forms are:

- *polyarticular JRA,* which affects many joints (usually five or more);

- *pauciarticular JRA,* which affects four or fewer joints; and
- *systemic JRA,* which affects both the joints and the internal organs.

Your physician can provide you with specific information on these three forms of JRA.

How is JRA diagnosed and treated?

Making a diagnosis of JRA is difficult since the signs and symptoms vary from child to child and there is no single test to diagnose the disease. In general, to make a diagnosis of JRA, the symptoms must have been present for six or more consecutive weeks.

There are several possible steps your physician may take to determine if your child has JRA. These include obtaining your child's health history by asking about symptoms and previous medical problems; conducting a physical examination to look for joint inflammation, rashes, nodules (small swollen lumps), and eye problems; requesting laboratory tests, which might support a diagnosis; ordering X-ray examinations to determine joint damage; and possibly obtaining a sample of fluid from a joint for examination.

Once the diagnosis of JRA has been made, your child's treatment program will be based on the symptoms and extent of the disease. The goals of any treatment program for JRA are to control inflammation, relieve pain, prevent or control joint damage, and maximize functional abilities. Your child's treatment program will usually include medications, exercise, and healthful eating practices. Other treatments, such as surgery, may be necessary for special problems. Because eye inflammation is sometimes associated with JRA, your child should get periodic eye examinations even when the JRA is inactive. If left untreated, eye problems associated with JRA can result in impaired vision.

3

Arthritis Medications

Appropriate medication, as suggested or prescribed by your physician, is an important component in the control of arthritis symptoms. These medications, like the other components of the treatment program, vary depending on the type and severity of the condition.

This chapter discusses nonsteroidal anti-inflammatory drugs (NSAIDs), corticosteroids, disease-modifying antirheumatic drugs (DMARDs), and other medications your physician may recommend to control the symptoms of your arthritis. Questions about the effectiveness of these medications and possible side effects will also be answered.

Your doctor will decide which medication may be right for you based on your medical history, a physical examination, and laboratory results. You may need to try several before finding the right one or the right combination. The doctor will want to know whether or not the medication is alleviating your symptoms and if you are experiencing any side effects. When taken properly under your doctor's supervision, medication—both prescription and over-the-counter—can be an effective tool in the successful management of arthritis symptoms.

What are NSAIDs?

NSAIDs, or nonsteroidal anti-inflammatory drugs, are a group of medications used to treat pain and inflammation. They must be used regularly in full doses to reduce the inflammation caused by diseases such as rheumatoid arthritis. If there is only a little inflammation, then an analgesic may be effective instead of an NSAID. When prescribing NSAIDs, or any other arthritis medication, physicians must consider the beneficial effects versus the potential side effects.

Aspirin, also known by the name acetylsalicylic acid or ASA, is the oldest NSAID. It is quite effective in relieving pain and inflammation. However, to achieve anti-inflammatory levels of aspirin in the blood, you may need to take two or three 300 mg tablets as often as four times a day, under the supervision of your doctor.

Although other NSAIDs work like aspirin, some are more potent and longer acting and so fewer pills are necessary to achieve the anti-inflammatory effect. These various NSAIDs come in the form of pills, suppositories, liquids, and injectables. Some are available by prescription only, while others are available over the counter.

How do I know if NSAIDs are right for me?

The best way to find out if NSAIDs may help you is by talking with your doctor. Although all NSAIDs are similar in action and side effects, some work better than others to treat certain types of arthritis and for certain people. You and your doctor will decide which drug and dosage are best for you depending on several factors—your overall health, age, the type of arthritis you have, and how you respond to the medication. If you're taking other medications while you are taking NSAIDs, this too can influence your physician's decision.

ALLERGY TIP

SIGNS OF AN ALLERGY TO THE MEDICINE YOU'RE TAKING INCLUDE:

- wheezing and difficulty breathing;
- hives, itching, skin rash or other skin problems; and/or
- puffiness in eyelids and around your eyes.

If you experience an allergic reaction, get to a hospital emergency room as soon as possible or call 911.

Do NSAIDs cause side effects?

A number of side effects are associated with the use of NSAIDs. Notable among these is irritation of the stomach, which may result in ulceration and bleeding. NSAIDs may also affect the kidneys, causing an increase in blood pressure and reducing kidney function. These side effects are more likely to occur in people over the age of 60 and in people with a history of peptic ulcer disease, kidney disease, or heart disease. Older people may also experience other side effects from NSAIDs, including mental confusion.

NSAIDs may also cause an abnormality of liver function, which is usually not serious and which can be detected with certain liver tests. NSAIDs may also interfere with the effectiveness of certain antihypertensive drugs and may increase a person's tendency to bleed when taken with anticoagulants (drugs used to prevent blood clots), such as warfarin sodium *(Coumadin)*. Drinking alcohol while taking NSAIDs may also increase the risk of side effects.

Aspirin may cause additional side effects, including ringing in the ears, dizziness, and potentially diminished hearing. These side effects are dose-related.

Aspirin is known to interfere with platelet function, increasing the tendency to bleed. This action is why aspirin is used to help prevent heart attacks and strokes, but people who have major bleeding problems should not take aspirin. Other NSAIDs interfere with platelet function but to a lesser degree. People may also develop allergic reactions to aspirin (and other NSAIDs), including nasal polyps (masses of swollen membranes), asthma, and sometimes hives.

Aspirin-like medications that have similar anti-inflammatory and pain-relieving properties but less adverse side effects on the stomach, kidneys, and platelets can be used. These are called nonacetylated salicylate preparations and are available by prescription. Salsalate *(Disalcid)* is one such aspirin-like medication.

The NSAIDs, including aspirin, are used to treat most types of arthritis. Your physician will decide whether over-the-counter NSAIDs or aspirin are appropriate or whether prescription NSAIDs might be more effective. The more potent NSAIDs, such as indomethacin *(Indocin)*, are used to control acute gout.

Which non-NSAID analgesics can be used to treat arthritis pain?

Acetaminophen may be helpful if you need just pain relief, are allergic to aspirin, or have had a peptic ulcer. The drug may provide relief from arthritis pain, but it does not affect inflammation, including the swelling of joints. It is

EXAMPLES OF PRESCRIPTION AND OTC NON-ASPIRIN NSAIDS*

GENERIC NAME	BRAND NAME
Diclofenac Sodium	Voltaren
Diclofenac Potassium	Cataflam
Diflunisal	Dolobid
Etodolac	Lodine
Fenoprofen Calcium	Nalfon
Flurbiprofen	Ansaid
Ibuprofen	Aches-N-Pain*, Advil*, Excedrin-IB*, Genpril*, Haltran*, Ibuprin*, Ibuprohm*, IbuTab*, Medipren*, Motrin, Midol 200*, Motrin-IB*, Nuprin*, PamprinIB*, Rufen, Saleto 200*, Trendar*
Indomethacin	Indocin
Ketoprofen	Orudis, Oruvail, Orudis KT*, Actron*
Meclofenamate Sodium	Meclomen
Nabumetone	Relafen
Naproxen	Naprosyn
Naproxen Sodium	Aflaxen, Anaprox, Aleve*
Oxaprozin	Daypro
Phenylbutazone	Butazolidin
Piroxicam	Feldene
Sulindac	Clinoril
Tolmetin Sodium	
Ketorolac	Tolectin
Tromethamine	Toradol

*Over-the-counter (OTC) medication

most commonly used to treat the pain of osteoarthritis. Acetaminophen is available without prescription. Familiar over-the-counter name-brand acetaminophen products include aspirin-free *Anacin, Bayer Select, Excedrin,* and *Tylenol.*

Acetaminophen may be associated with side effects in certain situations. It can aggravate liver damage if there is pre-existing damage or if the patient is abusing drugs or alcohol that are causing liver damage.

Tramadol hydrochloride *(Ultram)* is another type of non-NSAID that is used to treat arthritis pain. It is available only with a prescription and must be used under the direction of a physician.

Are narcotics ever used to treat arthritis pain?

Narcotics are strong painkillers that are prescribed only for a short time, such as following surgery or injury, such as a fracture, for example. Because arthritis is frequently a chronic, or long-term, condition, long-term use of narcotics can lead to addiction and has no effect on the inflammation causing the pain in the inflammatory types of arthritis. Examples of narcotics include codeine, morphine, propoxyphene *(Darvon)*, meperidine hydrochloride *(Demerol)*, hydromorphone hydrochloride *(Dilaudid)*, and hydrocodone *(Vicodin)*.

Is it true that I may be prescribed antidepressants to treat my arthritis and related musculoskeletal problems even if I'm not depressed?

Antidepressants can relieve chronic pain in people who are not necessarily depressed. They are taken in smaller doses than they would be for depression, however. These drugs work by blocking pain messengers in the brain. They can also help in bringing about more restful sleep patterns, which in turn may result in more effective pain management. Antidepressants are particularly helpful in treating fibromyalgia. Examples of antidepressants include amitriptyline *(Elavil)* and nortriptyline *(Pamelor)*.

Do muscle relaxants work well in the treatment of arthritis pain?

No. In general, muscle relaxants are not useful in treating arthritis. Muscle relaxants, however, such as cyclobenzaprine *(Flexeril)*, may be helpful in relieving the pain that accompanies fibromyalgia by decreasing muscle tension, which may aggravate the pain.

TYPES OF ASPIRIN AND OTHER SALICYLATES*

NON-PRESCRIPTION DRUG SALICYLATE	AMOUNT
Alka-Seltzer	324 mg aspirin
Anacin products	400 mg and 500 mg aspirin
Arthritis Pain Formula	500 mg aspirin
Arthropan*	870 mg choline salicylate
Ascriptin	325 mg aspirin
Aspergum	227.5 mg aspirin
Bayer products	325 mg, 500 mg and 650 mg (time release)
BC Powder	650 mg aspirin, 95 mg salicylamide
BC Powder Arthritis Strength	742 mg aspirin, 222 mg salicylamide
Bufferin products	324 mg, 486 mg and 500 mg aspirin
Cama Inlay Tabs	500 mg aspirin
Ecotrin products (enteric-coated)	325 mg and 500 mg aspirin
Empirin	325 mg aspirin
Excedrin	250 mg aspirin
Measurin	650 mg aspirin
Midol	454 mg aspirin
Mobigesic*	325 mg magnesium salicylate
Momentum	500 mg aspirin
P-A-C Compound	227 mg aspirin
Persistin	162.5 mg aspirin
Quiet World	227 mg aspirin
Trigesic	230 mg aspirin
St. Joseph's Aspirin for Children	81 mg aspirin
Vanquish Caplets	227 mg aspirin
Darvon Compound products	325 mg and 389 mg aspirin
Disalcid*	500 mg and 750 mg salsalate
Easprin	975 mg aspirin
Empirin #3	325 mg aspirin
Equagesic	325 mg aspirin
Fiorinal products	325 mg aspirin
Gemnisyn	325 mg aspirin
Magan*	545 mg magnesium salicylate
Percodan products	325 mg aspirin
Salflex*	500 mg and 750 mg salsalate
Supac	230 mg aspirin
Synalgos products	356.4 mg aspirin
Talwin Compound	325 mg aspirin
Trilisate products*	500 mg, 750 mg and 1,000 mg total salicylate
Zorprin	800 mg aspirin

*Non acetylated salicylates

What are corticosteroids?

Corticosteroids or glucocorticoids (cortisone, Prednisone) are often used to treat inflammatory forms of arthritis and related inflammatory conditions such as lupus. These medications are used in the treatment of arthritis for two reasons. First, they decrease inflammation and the damage it can cause, which is one of the goals of therapy for rheumatic diseases. Many people who have rheumatic diseases experience a lot of inflammation, which can take place in the joints (rheumatoid arthritis) or in various organs (lupus). One of the goals in the treatment of rheumatic diseases is to stop inflammation and the damage it causes. Second, corticosteroids are immunosuppressive, which means that they reduce the activity of the immune system. Rheumatoid arthritis and lupus are associated with abnormalities in the immune system. Examples of some brand-name corticosteroids are *Decadron, Cortone Acetate, Medrol, Prelone, Sterapred,* and *Deltasone.*

COMMONLY USED CORTICOSTEROIDS

TABLETS, PILLS	FOR LOCAL INJECTION
Cortisone	Aristocort
Decadron	Celestone
Delta-cortef	Cinalone
Deltasone	Depo-Medrol
Dexamethasone	Hydeltrasol
Hydrocortone	Hydeltra TBA
Kenacort	Kenalog
Medrol	
Methylprednisolone	
Orasone	
Prednisolone	
Prednisone	
Triamcinolone	

This is a partial list and includes generic and brand names. Various corticosteroid syrups are available for children.

Are corticosteroids the same as the steroids some athletes misuse?

Doctors sometimes refer to corticosteroids as steroids, but they should not be confused with the anabolic (muscle-building) steroid drugs that some athletes abuse. They are not the same. When taken as prescribed, corticosteroids can provide welcome relief from pain and inflammation.

Can side effects occur from corticosteroid use?

Corticosteroids can cause side effects and serious medical problems if used too long in high doses and not carefully monitored by a doctor. Most side effects are predictable and related to the dose.

Weight gain occurs when corticosteroids are used in higher doses. At first, most of the weight gain is from water retention only, but corticosteroids also increase body fat. The drugs will also increase your appetite, which can lead to further weight gain.

Some people find that corticosteroids cause them to have *mood swings*, ranging from feeling positive and uplifted to feeling sad, anxious, or depressed. The higher the dose, the more likely that these emotional effects will occur.

Nervousness may also occur, and difficulty sleeping while taking corticosteroids is common, especially if the dose is high and the medication is taken later in the day. In some instances, psychosis can occur. People with a history of serious mental health problems should consult their doctor about how to deal with these risks before taking corticosteroids.

CAUTION!

It is dangerous to suddenly stop or significantly reduce the amount of corticosteroids you are taking. Increasing the dose without instructions from your physician may be very harmful, even if you temporarily feel better. Always consult your physician before making any adjustments in the dose of Prednisone or other corticosteroid medications.

Taking higher doses of corticosteroids for more than a few weeks may cause mild weakness in arm or leg muscles, blurred vision, hair thinning or excessive hair growth, easy bruising of the skin, slow healing of cuts and wounds, acne, round face (moon face), slowed bone growth in children and adolescents, and osteoporosis (loss of bone calcium).

Occasional side effects associated with high-dose corticosteroid use for weeks or months include high blood pressure, elevated blood sugar, red or purple stretch marks on the skin, and stomach irritation or stomach ulcers, especially when the corticosteroids are taken with aspirin or NSAIDs. Corticosteroids can also worsen existing high blood pressure, diabetes, blood sugar problems, or ulcers. If you have had any of these conditions and need to take corticosteroids, it is very important to discuss this history with your doctor before beginning treatment.

What are some of the less common side effects of taking corticosteroids?

The less common side effects of taking corticosteroids for moderate or prolonged periods may include blurred vision from cataracts; glaucoma; avascular necrosis (a serious and painful condition that occurs most often in the hip when the bone is deprived of circulation); severe weakness of the muscles; and infections due to suppression of the immune system. The frequency and severity of the side effects from corticosteroids are related to the dose.

How effective are corticosteroids in the long run?

Corticosteroids may be helpful in controlling the joint symptoms of rheumatoid arthritis or lupus, as well as skin inflammations associated with lupus. Corticosteroids can be taken in low doses to control the symptoms of inflammatory forms of arthritis, resulting in fewer and less severe side effects.

What are DMARDs?

DMARDs, or disease-modifying anti-rheumatic drugs, are a group of drugs that can reduce the symptoms of rheumatoid arthritis, lupus, and perhaps other inflammatory forms of arthritis. They also have the potential to control the inflammation and limit the progression of the disease. They are usually taken with NSAIDs and frequently with low doses of corticosteroids. DMARDs are slower-acting, more powerful agents than NSAIDs. They work better when used early in the disease but may be helpful at any time during its course.

When would my doctor consider prescribing DMARDs?

Before recommending DMARD treatment, your doctor will consider how severe your disease is, how many joints are affected, which joints are affected, and how your arthritis has responded to other treatments. He or she will need to know about any other medical conditions you have that could make the use of DMARDs hazardous (for example, kidney disease or liver disease).

What is hydroxychloroquine?

Hydroxychloroquine is a DMARD that is effective in the treatment of such rheumatic diseases as rheumatoid arthritis and lupus. The drug helps relieve inflammation, swelling, stiffness, and joint pain. Its brand name is *Plaquenil*.

Is hydroxychloroquine a new medication?

No. This drug was originally developed to treat malaria, but it has also been used for many years to treat certain forms of inflammatory arthritis.

Hydroxychloroquine is usually used with NSAIDs and low doses of Prednisone. It is mainly used to reduce inflammation and possibly slow down the disease progression of rheumatoid arthritis. It is also used to reduce disease activity in lupus. Unlike other disease-modifying drugs used to treat rheumatic disorders, hydroxychloroquine does not increase the risk of infection, lower the number of white cells in the blood (which are needed to fight infection), or cause peptic ulcers.

How is hydroxychloroquine dispensed?

Hydroxychloroquine is available only by prescription. It is taken in tablet form, usually once or twice each day. People usually tolerate this medication well.

Are there any side effects of hydroxychloroquine?

Side effects can occur at any time during treatment and may include a bitter taste in the mouth, diarrhea, loss of appetite, nausea and vomiting, headache, dizziness, skin rash, and itching. These are generally minor and last for a very brief time. Most people have no side effects at all from hydroxychloroquine.

In rare instances, hydroxychloroquine may form deposits in the cornea (the transparent outer covering of the eye). You won't be able to tell they are there, although your ophthalmologist will be able to recognize them. They do not do any damage to the eyes and are not a reason to stop taking hydroxychloroquine.

In rare cases following prolonged or excessive use of hydroxychloroquine, the retina (the nerves in the back of the eye that enable you to see) could become injured. Early detection of this unusual occurrence can minimize damage. If this problem is detected, you will be asked to stop taking hydroxychloroquine. Your doctor will want you to have an eye examination before you begin taking hydroxychloroquine and then again every nine to twelve months while you continue to take it. In the rare event that you experience visual changes while taking the medication, call your doctor immediately.

What is methotrexate?

Methotrexate is a DMARD that decreases the activity and progression of rheumatoid arthritis and other conditions such as psoriatic arthritis (a condition that causes pain and swelling in some joints and scaly skin patches on some areas of the body). It has been the most effective drug used in treating RA for the last decade. Methotrexate was first developed to treat certain types of cancers and is used at much lower doses to treat rheumatic diseases. The drug has been studied for more than 25 years in the treatment of rheumatoid arthritis and in 1988 was approved by the Federal Drug Administration (FDA) for this use in adults. It is known by the brand name *Rheumatrex* but is also available in generic form.

How does methotrexate work?

Methotrexate decreases joint inflammation and alters the way the body uses folic acid, which is necessary for cell growth. Scientists suspect these actions account for the beneficial effect of methotrexate on patients with rheumatoid arthritis. Benefits include a decrease in the number of painful and swollen joints and in the progression of the disease. Methotrexate is usually taken with NSAIDs and frequently with low doses of Prednisone.

CAUTION!

Women on methotrexate must go off their medication during pregnancy and at least two to three months prior to a planned pregnancy! Methotrexate should not be taken by people who have serious kidney or liver disease, who drink alcohol or who have AIDS.

Does methotrexate relieve the symptoms of arthritis quickly?

Methotrexate may begin to work as early as three to six weeks after the beginning of treatment, but it can take as long as two to three months. The drug benefits a high percentage of people who take it and is well tolerated by most.

Doctors are increasingly prescribing methotrexate early in the course of RA to control inflammation before damage occurs, but it can be effective at any time during the course of the disease. If you have been on other medications and have not responded, methotrexate may be added or substituted for another medication later in the course of your illness.

How often would I take methotrexate?

Methotrexate is generally taken once a week, either orally (in pill or liquid form) or by injection. In some instances, your doctor may want you to take three consecutive doses 12 hours apart over the course of two days. More frequent use can be associated with serious side effects.

You will generally be advised to take the medication on the same day each week and to keep calendar records of the doses you take. If you should happen to forget when you last took a dose of methotrexate, you should call your doctor and explain the situation. If you miss a dose, do not take the missed dose, and do not double the next one. Call your doctor, explain the circumstances, and follow his or her advice.

What are the most common side effects of methotrexate?

The most common side effects are upset stomach, nausea, vomiting, loss of appetite, diarrhea, and mouth sores. If these side effects occur while you are taking methotrexate, contact your doctor. A change in the dose or in how you take your methotrexate can usually ease the side effects. Some of the side effects may be decreased or eliminated by taking folic acid.

What are some of the rarer side effects of methotrexate?

In rare cases, methotrexate has been known to cause liver damage. If you take the medication, your physician will monitor your liver function to detect any possible damage. It is vitally important that you not harm your liver in any other way while you are on methotrexate, particularly by drinking alcohol. Your physician will monitor your liver function by doing blood liver tests while you are on the medication.

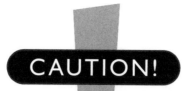

CAUTION!

If you miss a dose of your methotrexate, do not take the missed dose and do not double the next dose. Just continue your regular dosing schedule and check with your doctor.

In rare situations, methotrexate may affect the lungs. If you experience such problems as shortness of breath, fever, or a cough while taking methotrexate, contact your physician immediately.

Are there any other special considerations regarding taking methotrexate?

Regular laboratory tests are absolutely necessary while taking methotrexate. Before you receive this medication, standard tests will be done, and once therapy starts, testing will be done every one to two months. Blood tests will be performed on a regular basis to monitor your liver and bone marrow for changes. It is important that you keep your scheduled laboratory and doctor's appointments so that side effects can be identified early and your medication stopped or the dose modified to alleviate problems.

What is sulfasalazine used for?

Sulfasalazine *(Azulfidine)* is a DMARD that has the ability to slow the progression of the joint destruction associated with rheumatoid arthritis. Like other DMARDs, sulfasalazine is frequently used with NSAIDs and low doses of Prednisone. It may also be added to other DMARDs for better control of arthritis. Common side effects include nausea and diarrhea. Occasionally, skin rashes occur. Sulfasalazine is given in pill form, usually two to four times a day. It is important to take sulfasalazine in evenly-divided doses, preferably after meals, over a 24-hour period.

What is gold treatment?

Gold is another DMARD. Some brand-name examples of gold are *Solganal* (aurothioglucose) and *Ridaura* (auranofin). Gold treatment is prescribed for people with rheumatoid arthritis, juvenile rheumatoid arthritis, or psoriatic arthritis.

Gold treatment works slowly and gradually; most people begin to notice a decrease in their stiffness, joint pain, and swelling two to six months after they start the treatment. Some people receiving gold treatment actually go into remission, but for most, it reduces active swelling of the joints. For many people, gold works for two or three years then loses its effectiveness.

How is gold administered?

Gold can be either injected into a muscle (as with *Solganal*) or taken in capsule form, known as oral gold (auranofin or *Ridaura)*. Oral gold is not as effective as injectable gold, which must be administered by a qualified professional.

If you are prescribed injectable gold, you will begin with a small dose to make sure you don't have a reaction to it. Every week you'll receive larger amounts until the full dose is reached. The frequency of doses is then adjusted depending on how your arthritis improves and on whether you have any side effects. Your doctor will see you regularly and check you blood and urine for side effects.

What are some of the side effects of gold treatment?

Most of the side effects are minor, but some can be serious. Side effects can occur at any time during treatment, and they may persist for several months after patients stop taking the gold. Side effects of injectable gold treatment include rash, mouth sores, a metallic taste, protein in the urine, and lowering of the white blood count. The major side effect of oral gold is diarrhea.

Less common side effects from gold treatment include liver, intestinal, and lung damage. These problems have been reported in people treated with gold but are quite rare.

How effective are topical pain relievers?

Topical pain relievers temporarily relieve the pain of arthritis, in particular, osteoarthritis. They include creams, rubs, or sprays that are put on the skin overlying a painful muscle or joint. Creams containing capsaicin (cap-sa-shun), such as *Dolorac* and *Zostrix,* may be used alone or with other medications to temporarily relieve joint pain. Capsaicin decreases the ability of nerve endings in the skin to sense pain. Other creams, such as *BenGay*, contain methyl salicylate, which also eases arthritis pain.

When are joint injections used to treat arthritis?

If a physician does not know what is causing the swelling of a joint, he or she may decide to aspirate the joint with a needle and syringe to obtain and analyze joint fluid. This is done using a sterile technique after the skin and tissues are anesthetized. The joint fluid may be analyzed for the number of white blood cells present, for infection, and for the presence of crystals. This information will help the doctor decide if the swelling is caused by an infection, inflammation (such as gout) or osteoarthritis. In some cases when only one joint is affected, the doctor may inject the joint with a cortisone preparation, such as methylprednisolone acetate *(Depo-Medrol),* triamcinolone hexacetonide *(Aristospan),* or triamcinolone diacetate *(Aristocort)* to temporarily relieve the pain and inflammation.

How is gout treated?

In addition to the more potent NSAIDs, colchicine is used to treat acute gouty arthritis. Colchicine is not an NSAID but a different type of anti-inflammatory drug that inhibits the functioning of white blood cells called polymorphonuclear leukocytes, which are active players in the inflammation of gout. Colchicine is taken in tablet form. If you have an acute attack of gout, your physician may prescribe up to six tablets to be taken over a 24-hour period. Colchicine may also be taken in low doses for months after an acute attack to reduce the likelihood of future attacks.

WHAT YOU SHOULD ASK ABOUT YOUR MEDICATIONS

- What is its name?
- How much do I take?
- How and when do I take it?
- How long will it be before it works?
- What benefits can I expect?
- When should I contact my doctor if I don't get relief?
- What side effects should I watch for?
- What other drugs should I not take with it?

Because colchicine can cause side effects, it must be taken only under the supervision of a physician who is experienced and knowledgeable in its use and after he or she has given you careful instructions. The most frequent side effects are nausea, vomiting, and diarrhea.

Allopurinol *(Lopurin, Zyloprim)* is used to prevent attacks of gout and to inhibit the accumulation of uric acid or urate deposits in tissues (joints, skin, and kidneys). The side effects of allopurinol include skin rashes and, uncommonly, liver injury.

Probenecid *(Benemid)* is another drug used to prevent attacks of gout and the accumulation of urate deposits. It acts by increasing the excretion of uric acid by the kidneys. The side effects include nausea, vomiting, and skin rashes.(See page 24 for more about the treatment of gout.)

What are some good tips on how to use arthritis medications safely?

It is important to try to discuss any concerns you have about the medications prescribed for you with your doctor. Your goal should be to gain as many positive results from your medication as possible, with as few side effects as possible. Your doctor is also looking for a positive outcome. Follow your doctor's instructions on the use of your medications and if you're ever in doubt, ask questions until you feel you have gotten satisfactory answers. Being actively involved in the management of your disease will bring you positive results. Your doctor is your best professional resource when it comes to your health.

Common questions that you should ask your physician about your medication include the following:
- What is its name?
- How much should I take?
- How and when should I take it?
- Are there any precautions I should know about, such as taking my medication with food?
- How long will it be before my medication works?
- What benefits can I expect?
- How soon should I contact you if I don't get relief?
- What side effects should I be watching for?
- What other drugs should not be taken with the one you have prescribed?

Be sure your physician knows all the medicines you are taking, including over-the-counter drugs.

TIPS FOR SAFE MEDICATION USE

- Take your medicines exactly as your doctor instructs.
- Do not skip a dose unless your doctor recommends it.
- Don't stop taking a medicine unless your doctor recommends it.
- Keep in mind that it takes some medications longer to work than others.

I've taken my medication for a while and I feel better. Can I stop using it?

It is important to take your medication exactly as your physician prescribes. Do not decrease or increase your dosage unless specifically instructed by your doctor to do so. Beginning to feel better means that your medication is working well to control your arthritis, and you want to continue that progress. Stopping your medication without your physician's advice could result in the return of inflammation and, in some cases, serious complications. Your arthritis pain may be gone while you are taking your medication, but the arthritis itself is not necessarily gone. You should always consult with your physician before adjusting your medication therapy.

If I feel worse after taking medication for a while, should I stop taking it?

Keep your doctor apprised of how you feel. If you experience side effects, call your doctor immediately—the doctor needs to know this information. Your dose or the type of medication you are taking can be changed once the doctor is made aware of problems.

What will happen if I take just a few extra pills?

Taking a few extra pills is not a good idea at all. It's tempting to want to take more medicine or to try unhealthy remedies, such as drinking alcohol, to escape your pain. But by doing this, you may create very serious problems for yourself.

4

Other Treatments for Arthritis

Research studies often suggest that a positive state of mind increases our capacity to heal. Taking a proactive stance by "helping yourself" can motivate you to be more in control of the physical and emotional components of arthritis. In this chapter you will read about the benefits of massage therapy, relaxation techniques, heat and cold treatments, and assistive devices. As with any treatment for arthritis, these techniques should be undertaken with advice from your physician, physical therapist, or occupational therapist.

Many of the techniques discussed here are spiritually uplifting and relaxing, leading to a very real reduction in pain. Using these and other methods allows you to take charge of your circumstances and helps you to manage your arthritis effectively. Your doctor may be able to provide you with more information about the connection between emotional and physical well-being.

Are there items or devices available that will make my life with arthritis easier?

Yes, there are, and they may be necessary if arthritis is severely impairing your function. Assistive devices are products or aids that protect injured joints from further damage. There are three types of assistive devices:

- Products that allow you to carry out routine activities, such as bathing, cleaning, and dressing. Examples include grab bars in the bathroom, large-handled utensils for eating, and aids for fastening and unfastening clothing.

- Aids that improve mobility, keep joints from becoming too stiff, and distribute weight over a number of joints. Examples include canes and walkers.
- Devices that help stabilize joints, provide strength, and reduce pain and inflammation. Examples include braces and splints.

What effect do heat or cold treatments have on arthritis symptoms?

The application of heat or cold is a method of noninvasive treatment that can gently ease the pain and stiffness of arthritis. Using heat or cold treatments on achy joints may give you the short-term relief you are looking for. Heat or cold are commonly used along with medication, joint protection, rest, and other pain management methods.

What happens when I use heat or cold treatments?

Heat treatments relax your muscles and stimulate circulation. They are particularly effective before or after exercise. Cold treatments numb the area so you don't feel as much pain. You may need to experiment to find which method works best for you.

What methods of heat and cold treatments are available?

Both heat and cold treatments are available in various forms. You can use dry heat, such as a heating pad, an electric blanket, or a heat lamp. Good moist methods include baths, whirlpool dips, and hydrocollator packs.

For cold treatments, you can use ice or cold packs. In a pinch, even bags of frozen vegetables, with a towel as a buffer between the ice and your skin, work well.

These treatments may be easy, but it's important to use heat and cold safely. Don't use either treatment for more than 20 minutes at a time unless otherwise instructed by your doctor. Let your skin return to normal temperature between applications. Don't use heat with penetrating rubs or creams—their use together can result in skin burns.

Protect the skin over any bone that is close to the surface of the skin by placing padding over the area. This will help guard against burning or freezing.

I've heard that massage may be helpful to someone with arthritis. Is it?

Massage brings warmth to sore areas and is soothing. You can massage your own muscles or you can ask your doctor to recommend a professional

HOT AND COOL TIPS

- Soak in a warm bath, shower, Jacuzzi or whirlpool.
- Place a heating pad on the painful area.
- Don't sleep with the heating pad on. You might burn yourself.
- Use an electric blanket or mattress pad. Turn it up before you get out of bed to combat morning stiffness.
- Use flannel sheets. They feel warmer against your skin.
- Use a hot water bottle wrapped in a towel to keep your feet, back or hands warm.
- Before getting dressed, warm your clothes by placing them in the dryer for a few minutes.
- Place hot packs on the painful area. Don't let the pack get too hot, and always provide towel layering between the hot pack and your skin.

- Place a cold pack or ice bag on the painful area. You can buy these at the drugstore, or you can make one by wrapping a towel around a bag of frozen vegetables.

who is trained to give massages. Be sure to tell your massage therapist that you have arthritis and point out your tender areas.

When giving yourself a massage, use lotion or oil to help your hands glide over your skin. Ask your physical therapist or consult one of the many books available on the subject to learn effective self-massage techniques.

How does ultrasound work?

Ultrasound is a technique in which high-energy sound waves are used to comfort painful joints and muscles. A physical or occupational therapist must perform this technique.

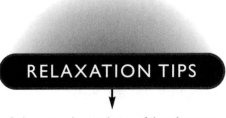

RELAXATION TIPS

↓

Pick a quiet place and time of day when you
won't be disturbed for at least 15 minutes.

↓

Make yourself as comfortable as possible
before beginning. Loosen any tight clothing and
uncross your legs, ankles and arms. Sit in a comfortable chair or lie down. Try to practice relaxation daily. If you can't practice this often, set
aside a time for it at least four times a week.

↓

Don't expect immediate results. It may
be several weeks before you notice
results from some techniques.

↓

Remember that relaxation should be
helpful. If these techniques are unpleasant
to you or make you more nervous
and anxious, stop. You may manage your
stress better with other techniques.

Why are relaxation techniques recommended for people with arthritis?

People who are in pain experience both physical and emotional stress.
Pain and stress both have similar effects on the body. Muscles become tight,
and breathing becomes fast and shallow. Heart rate and blood pressure go up.
Relaxation can help you reverse these effects. It gives you a sense of control
and well-being and makes it easier to manage pain.

Relaxation may not come easily, especially if you are in pain. It takes
practice. The best time to use relaxation skills to manage pain is before the
pain becomes too intense. A number of techniques used to achieve mental
relaxation are described in Chapter 7.

There is no best way to learn how to relax. Everyone responds differently to various techniques. The important thing to remember is to relax both your body and your mind.

How is biofeedback used?

Biofeedback is most commonly used in the treatment of fibromyalgia. It involves the use of sensitive electrical equipment to help you become more aware of your body's reaction to stress and pain and to learn how to control your body's physical reactions. The equipment monitors your heart rate, blood pressure, skin temperature, and muscle tension. These body signals are shown on a computer screen or gauge so you can see how your body is reacting.

Biofeedback helps you learn how your body reacts when your muscles are tense or relaxed. If you practice a relaxation technique while using the equipment, you can learn to control some of your body's responses to pain. One advantage of biofeedback is that it shows you that you have the ability to relax; it's just a matter of learning how.

5

Pain Management

Pain can be the most difficult part of having an arthritis-related condition, but not only is pain management possible, it can be highly effective. In this chapter you will learn about the reasons for and causes of arthritis pain, how people react to pain, and, most important, how to manage pain.

Because the pain of arthritis is triggered by inflammation in the joint or deterioration of cartilage in the joint, it is important to take your medications exactly as prescribed by your physician. At the same time, you should recognize that other factors contribute to the pain of arthritis. Overusing your affected joint will make the pain worse, so you should always practice joint-protection techniques (see Chapter 10). And if the muscles surrounding the joint are weak, strain on the joint will result in more pain, so it is important to do regular exercise to increase and maintain muscle strength.

Feeling worried, anxious, depressed, or stressed can magnify pain. You can overcome some of these feelings by sharing your fears, frustrations, and experiences. A good place in which to do this is a group setting where others are trying to cope with the same challenges of living with arthritis. By sharing, you'll be exposed to new ideas for coping with pain and realize that others are experiencing the same pain as you are.

What causes my arthritis pain?

Just as there are different types of arthritis, there are different types of pain. Someone with the same type of arthritis as you have may feel a different kind of pain. Even your own pain may vary from day to day.

Arthritis pain is caused by:
- *Inflammation of the joint lining*—the process that causes the redness and swelling in your joints
- *Damage to joint cartilage*—a result of injury, deterioration, or inflammation
- *Muscle strain*—the result when overworked muscles are trying to protect your joints from painful movements

What function, if any, does pain serve?

Pain is your body's alarm system. It tells you something is wrong. When part of your body is injured or hurt, nerves in that area release chemical signals. Other nerves send those signals to your brain, where they are recognized as pain. Pain is often your body's way of telling you that you need to do something. For example, if you touch a hot stove, pain signals from your brain make you pull your hand away. This type of pain helps to protect you.

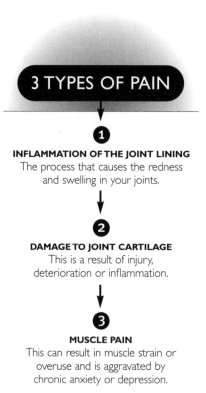

3 TYPES OF PAIN

①

INFLAMMATION OF THE JOINT LINING
The process that causes the redness
and swelling in your joints.

②

DAMAGE TO JOINT CARTILAGE
This is a result of injury,
deterioration or inflammation.

③

MUSCLE PAIN
This can result in muscle strain or
overuse and is aggravated by
chronic anxiety or depression.

What can I do to manage my pain?

Your physician should have you on the appropriate medications for your condition. Take your medication as prescribed. Your doctor and members of your health-care team will recommend other treatments you can do on your own to help manage your pain and move more easily.

Treatments for arthritis pain can be divided into several categories: medication, exercise, heat/cold, pacing (developing a comfortable pattern for your daily schedule), joint protection, surgery, and self-help skills. There are things you can do in each of these areas to help yourself feel better and move easier. See Chapter 3 and 4 for more information.

What are some helpful mental techniques I can use to control my pain?

Develop a wellness attitude. Arthritis can limit you, but it doesn't have to control you. One way to reduce your pain is to build your life around wellness, not pain and sickness. Continue to enjoy the things you've always loved, rather than focusing on lost abilities.

Try not to dwell on your pain. The amount of time you spend focusing on your pain has a great deal to do with how much discomfort you feel. People who dwell on their pain say that it is worse than those who don't—mind over matter therefore has merit! Redirect your thoughts by focusing on things that make you feel good. Develop a hobby, involve yourself in helping others, pursue new interests, try activities that you've always wanted to do.

Practice positive self-talk. Are there days when you wake up, get out of bed, and feel a smile creasing your face from ear to ear even before you brush your teeth? You know immediately that it's going to be a terrific day. If you can tap into your reserves of that kind of positive energy on a regular basis, you will be in a good position to motivate yourself past your pain. It may seem odd at first to talk to yourself about your own attitudes and behaviors, but you'll discover that it can make a difference. The best part is you'll always have the last word!

6

Overcoming Fatigue

From time to time, everyone experiences the exhaustion and overall lack of energy characteristic of fatigue, but with some arthritis-related conditions, this fatigue can be unrelenting and debilitating. This chapter will help you understand what causes arthritis-related fatigue and give you some practical advice for managing it.

Fatigue is a very real medical symptom, which can have a significant impact on your overall quality of life. The fact that you feel fatigued may indicate that your disease is not adequately controlled. Don't hesitate to discuss your fatigue with your doctor or other members of your health-care team.

What is fatigue?

Fatigue is a feeling of tiredness or exhaustion that can make performing tasks difficult. It can range from mild tiredness at the end of a busy day to a chronic feeling of exhaustion that never seems to lift.

Fatigue affects everyone individually—at different times and in different ways. You may feel tired, as if you have no energy; this is often compared with the tired feeling that you might have with the flu. Fatigue may also increase your pain and make you feel a loss of control, a lack of concentration, or just plain irritable.

What does fatigue have to do with arthritis?

Fatigue is a frequent symptom of many arthritis-related conditions, such as rheumatoid arthritis and lupus, and a major symptom of fibromyalgia. There are many factors that can bring about fatigue. These causes can be broken down into three primary areas—physical, emotional, and environmental.

What are some of the physical causes contributing to fatigue?

The disease process itself may bring about fatigue, especially in conditions that involve systemic inflammation, such as rheumatoid arthritis and lupus. Some people with arthritis may also have other illnesses, which can contribute to fatigue. Anemia—whether related to arthritis or to other causes—can also result in fatigue. Each of these physical causes must be specifically treated, so be sure to discuss your fatigue with your doctor.

Other physical factors that can cause or aggravate fatigue include poor sleep patterns and too little physical activity.

What are some of the emotional causes of fatigue?

Living day to day with any chronic disease or chronic pain problem can be emotionally draining. This can take a toll on you and lead to increased bouts of fatigue. Associated anxiety and depression, overextending yourself, and trying to hide the illness from others can also bring about fatigue.

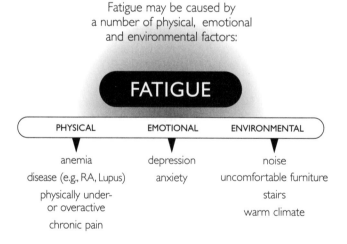

Fatigue may be caused by a number of physical, emotional and environmental factors:

FATIGUE

PHYSICAL	EMOTIONAL	ENVIRONMENTAL
anemia	depression	noise
disease (e.g., RA, Lupus)	anxiety	uncomfortable furniture
physically under- or overactive		stairs
chronic pain		warm climate

What are some of the environmental factors that can contribute to fatigue?

Any factor that makes your environment less comfortable or more difficult to navigate can contribute to your fatigue. Such factors could include loud noises, extreme temperatures or temperature changes, uncomfortable furniture, having to navigate many stairs, long commutes in heavy traffic, and long waits, to name a few.

What are some of the ways I can manage my fatigue?

Just as there are many causes of fatigue, there are many approaches to managing it. If your inflammatory arthritis is a major component of the fatigue, appropriate medications are necessary. In addition, you may need to become more proficient at saving your energy, become more aware of your body, and learn to strike a better balance between rest and activity. Eliminate or reduce energy-draining activities when possible. Whether you are managing a corporation or your personal well-being, planning makes sense.

What steps do I need to take to put together a self-management plan?

Look at all the tasks you do at home and at work during a normal day and week. Cross off anything that isn't necessary, and delegate some of the remaining tasks to others. Involve your family—you'll be amazed at how many things on your "to do" list that you thought were essential really aren't!

Make a daily schedule and assess the amount of time required for each task and how tiring those tasks might be, and schedule in rest breaks. Combine chores and errands so you can get more things done with less effort. Shortcuts are definitely an option! Prepare meals in advance. Sit often, and take as many short rest breaks as possible. Use labor-saving devices, such as an electric garage door opener, a microwave oven, and a food processor. Use self-help devices, such as tools with enlarged handles and jar openers, to help make jobs easier.

What role does sleep play in fatigue?

Getting a good night's sleep restores your energy and helps you cope with pain. It also gives your joints a chance to rest. Even a nap during the day may be just what you need to restore your energy and lift your spirits.

What can I do to get a better night's sleep?

Maintain a regular daily schedule of activities; exercise, but not too late and not too strenuously in the evening; try to relax one hour before bedtime; make your bedroom as quiet and comfortable as possible; try waking up at the same time every day, even on weekends and holidays; avoid caffeine (in coffee, tea, cocoa, and some soft drinks) or alcohol before bedtime; take a warm bath before going to bed; listen to soothing music or a relaxation tape. If you continue to have trouble sleeping, talk with your doctor. When a sleep disturbance is treated, the level of fatigue usually diminishes.

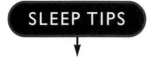

SLEEP TIPS

Maintain a regular daily schedule of activities.

Exercise, but not late in the evening.

Set aside a time in the evening for relaxation, such as an hour before bedtime.

Make your bedroom as quiet and comfortable as possible.

Go to bed and arise at the same time every day, even on weekends and holidays.

Avoid caffeine (in coffee, tea, cocoa, some soft drinks) or alcohol before bedtime.

Take a warm bath before going to bed.

Listen to soothing music or a relaxation tape.

Is it true that exercise can actually help alleviate the symptoms of fatigue?

Many people think that exercising will reduce their energy, but usually just the opposite is true. Engaging in the right type and right amount of exercise helps keep your muscles strong and bones healthy. A good exercise program also helps you keep or restore flexibility. Exercise can improve your sense of well-being and may result in an overall increase in energy. (For more about exercise and arthritis, see Chapter 8.) Before beginning any exercise program, consult with your doctor and physical or occupational therapist. To be effective, the exercise must be tailored to you and your type of arthritis.

Is following my treatment plan really important in warding off fatigue?

Following the treatment plan you and your physician have designed is the best way to avoid problems with fatigue. Don't skip medications or exercises on the days you feel good. This can backfire and lead to increased symptoms. Fatigue may be a sign of increased disease activity or inflammation. Report any increase in fatigue or general changes in your condition to your doctor so appropriate measures can be taken.

I really dislike asking for assistance when I'm fatigued. Why is this helpful?

Asking for assistance when you are fatigued may prevent you from becoming overextended, and as a result, triggering a flare. Don't be afraid to ask for help when you need it. Be honest about your limitations. Talk with family and friends about your fatigue, your need to rest, and how they can help. Family, friends, and co-workers would rather help you than have you be confined to bed. Also, seek help from your health-care provider, who is trained to help you manage your disease or condition and the resulting fatigue.

Attending support groups for people with arthritis can provide you with emotional assistance in managing your condition. Listening to and learning from a group of peers who are experiencing the same feelings and symptoms as you are can be very helpful.

7

Dealing with Stress

As if life weren't already stressful enough, having a chronic disease can add a whole layer of stress to your life. By learning how to deal with your stress in a positive manner, you can reduce pain, feel healthier, and manage your disease more effectively.

One of the best ways to cope with stress is by learning to truly relax. Relaxation is more than just sitting back, reading, or watching television. It is a state of calm in which you are in control of your body and mind. This chapter details several stress management/relaxation techniques, such as deep breathing, progressive relaxation, and guided imagery.

What is stress?

Stress is a state of heightened bodily or mental tension. Too much stress can increase pain and make it harder for you to deal with the challenges of arthritis or other chronic diseases.

Stressful events are not only what you might consider "negative" occasions. Weddings, births, and vacations are happy events, but they can be very stressful. Dealing with all kinds of stress is a daily challenge because stress is a normal part of life.

What are the signs of stress?

The most common signs of stress are tiredness/exhaustion; muscle tension; anxiety; irritability/anger; nervousness/trembling; sleeplessness; cold, sweaty hands; a loss of or an increase in appetite; grinding teeth/clenching jaws; or general physical discomfort (weakness, dizziness, headache, or pain in the back or muscles).

Some of these symptoms may stem from problems other than stress, such as having the flu or experiencing increased inflammatory disease activity. You should tell your doctor during your visits if you experience symptoms that you believe are stress-related. If you and your doctor determine that stress is contributing to the problem, you can work together to evaluate your situation and try to change it.

How are people with chronic diseases affected by stress?

People with rheumatic conditions go through stressful periods, just as everyone else does, but having a chronic disease can mean there are additional challenges to deal with and adjustments to make. For people with conditions such as fibromyalgia, stress may be a major factor in perpetuating their pain and poor sleep patterns. Chances are that you will need to make changes in your lifestyle and rely more on family members and health-care professionals to help keep your levels of stress under control.

Does stress cause arthritis?

No, it doesn't, but stress can have a negative effect on your body, which can magnify your arthritis symptoms. Taking good care of your body can help you build up resistance to stress. There are many ways to do this. These include eating a balanced diet; exercising; getting enough rest and sleep; using energy-saving techniques, such as pacing your activities and scheduling rest periods; and attempting to incorporate positive activities into your life and eliminating negative influences.

What happens when I am stressed?

When you feel stressed, your body becomes tense. If the stress is chronic, this tension can increase the pain in your muscles. This increased pain may make you feel helpless, and you may also become depressed because of your limited abilities. A cycle of stress, pain, limited/lost abilities, and depression may develop. This is particularly true if you have fibromyalgia. If you make an effort to understand how your body reacts physically and emotionally to stress, and then how to manage it, you can help break that destructive cycle.

What are some of the physical changes triggered by stress?

Some of your body's reactions to stress are easy to predict. At stressful times, the body releases chemicals into your bloodstream. As a result, your

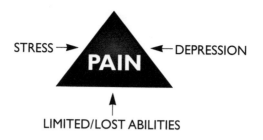

STRESS → PAIN ← DEPRESSION

↑
LIMITED/LOST ABILITIES

Stress, depression and
limited/lost abilities can
all contribute to pain.

heart beats faster, your breathing rate increases, your blood pressure increases, and your muscles become more tense.

When stress is handled in a positive way, the body restores itself to normal. At times, however, you may be unable to deal with stress constructively. As a result, stress-related tension builds up and, with no outlet, takes a toll on your body. This buildup of stress can take many forms—you may have headaches, an upset stomach, or a disease flare. Stress also affects the immune system, but it is not known exactly how diseases like arthritis are affected by this connection.

What are some of the emotional changes triggered by stress?

Your mind's reaction to stress is harder to predict than your physical reactions. Your emotional reactions are all your own, varying from situation to situation and depending on what else is going on in your life at that moment. These reactions may include feelings of fear, anxiety, helplessness, loss of control, annoyance, or frustration.

Small amounts of stress actually help when we need to perform our best—during an exam, an athletic event, or on stage, for example. Too much stress, though, can make some people accident-prone, more likely to make mistakes, or unable to perform at all.

What causes stress?

What causes you the most worry and concern? What situations make you feel anxious, nervous, or afraid? Learning what causes you stress is a personal discovery. Once you know, you can decide how best to modify those aspects of your life in an effort to decrease your stress levels. The ideal is to reach the point where you can stop yourself when you feel your body or mind becoming overly stressed. Keep a diary or chart if you can, and record the causes of your stress as well as any physical or emotional symptoms you experience. This will help you learn to recognize the signs of stress and begin to manage them.

How can I change or eliminate stress?

Once you've identified the causes of your stress, divide them into those causes that you can do something about and those you can't. Focus on what can be changed, and try to make changes in those areas of your life. Reduce as many hassles of daily life as you can: Avoid high-traffic areas on your way to work whenever possible, or take advantage of flex-time to leave earlier or later for work. Set your alarm clock a little earlier to avoid having to rush. Make a list of priorities: What needs to be done now? What can be postponed? What can be eliminated? You may need to buy groceries today, but the laundry can wait until tomorrow. And perhaps the lawn can wait until next week.

SAMPLE STRESS DIARY

DATE	CAUSE OF STRESS	TIME	PHYSICAL SYMPTOMS	EMOTIONAL SYMPTOMS
4/18	getting kids off to school	7am	fast heartbeat, tightness of neck	feel rushed, disorganized
4/18	stuck in traffic	8:30 am	headache, heart beating faster, legs aching	frustrated, angry at being late
4/18	meeting presentation	10 am	fast heartbeat, dry throat, clammy palms	anxious, nervous

Keep a diary or chart if you can and record the causes of your stress as well as physical or emotional symptoms you experience. Keeping a stress diary can help you learn what causes your stress and how you can avoid it.

QUESTIONS USED TO DO A REALITY CHECK

LEARN TO PUT STRESSFUL SITUATIONS IN
PERSPECTIVE BY ASKING THESE QUESTIONS:

- Does this situation reflect a threat signaling harm, or a challenge signaling an opportunity?
- Are there other ways to look at this situation?
- What exactly is at stake?
- What are you saying to yourself right now?
- What are you afraid will occur?
- How do you know this will happen?
- What evidence do you have that this will happen?
- Is there evidence that contradicts this conclusion?
- What coping resources are available to you?

What if there is something that I have no control over that just always causes stress?

If you can't change the situation, change your outlook. Realize that you can only change yourself, not other people. Some situations cannot be changed, so you have to learn to deal effectively with them. Try to "roll with the punches." Being flexible will help you keep a positive attitude in spite of the challenges.

Can deep breathing help reduce stress?

Yes, it can. Sit in a comfortable chair with your feet on the floor, your arms at your sides, and your eyes closed. Breathe in, saying to yourself, "I am . . ." then breathe out saying ". . . relaxed." Continue breathing slowly, silently repeating something soothing to yourself such as, "My hands . . . are warm; my feet . . . are warm; my breathing is deep and smooth; my heartbeat . . . is calm and steady; I feel calm . . . and at peace." Always coordinate the words with your breathing.

Does muscle relaxation help reduce stress?

Yes, muscle relaxation is one of the most common forms of stress management. Close your eyes and take a deep breath. Hold your breath for a few seconds and breathe out, letting your stress flow out with your breath. Let all your muscles feel heavy, and let your whole body sink into the surface beneath you. Beginning with your feet and calves, slowly tense your muscles. Hold for several seconds, then release and relax the muscles. Slowly work your way through your body using the same technique. Continue breathing deeply. Enjoy the feeling of being completely relaxed for a few minutes before opening your eyes.

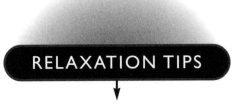

RELAXATION TIPS

Pick a quiet place and time of day when you
won't be disturbed for at least 15 minutes.

Make yourself as comfortable as possible before
beginning. Loosen any tight clothing and uncross
your legs, ankles and arms. Sit in a comfortable
chair or lie down. Try to practice relaxation daily.
If you can't practice this often, set aside a time
for it at least four times a week.

↓

Don't expect immediate results. It may
be several weeks before you notice
results from some techniques.

↓

Remember that relaxation should be
helpful. If these techniques are unpleasant
to you or make you more nervous
and anxious, stop. You may manage your
stress better with other techniques.

How do guided imagery and visualization help reduce stress?

Guided imagery is similar to a guided daydream. It helps you divert your attention, refocusing your mind away from your stress. Close your eyes, take a deep breath and hold it for several seconds. Breathe out slowly, feeling your body relax as you do. Think about a place you have been where you felt pleasure and comfort. Imagine it in as much detail as possible—how it looks, smells, sounds, and feels. Recapture the positive feelings you had then, and keep them in your mind. Take several deep breaths and enjoy feeling relaxed and peaceful before opening your eyes.

Visualization (also called vivid imagery) is similar to guided imagery. It allows you to imagine yourself any way you want, doing what you like to do. Visualization can be used for an extended period of time or while you are involved in other activities.

In one form of visualization, you remember pleasant scenes from your past or create new scenes in your mind. Another form of visualization involves thinking of symbols that represent the pain or stress in different parts of your body.

What are some common methods of relaxation that I could try?

Prayer or meditation is very relaxing and comforting for some people. You may want to make a tape recording of a soothing inspirational message or practice your own type of personal prayer.

Relaxation audiotapes and videotapes can help guide you through the relaxation process. These tapes instruct you in how to relax so you don't have to concentrate on remembering the directions. Many professional tapes are available for purchase. You might also want to make your own tape of your favorite relaxation routine.

8

Exercise and Arthritis

For many years it was thought that people with arthritis should not exercise because it would damage their joints. Now doctors and therapists know that exercise can actually improve the health and fitness of people with arthritis without hurting their joints. Exercise helps keep your joints moving, keeps the muscles around your joints strong, keeps bone and cartilage tissue strong and healthy, improves your ability to go about daily activities, and improves your overall health and fitness.

When you incorporate exercise into your daily routine, accepting it as a way of life, exercise can also decrease depression, improve self-esteem, and give you a better sense of well-being.

This chapter elaborates on the benefits of exercise for people who have arthritis and will help you get started on an exercise program. It also discusses exercises that are recommended for people with arthritis and how to get the greatest benefits from exercise.

How does exercise help in the management of my arthritis?

Along with medications, rest, and the other aspects of your treatment program, regular exercise can help keep your joints in working order so that you can continue your daily activities. Exercise may also help prevent further joint damage. Exercise is good for you because it keeps your bones and muscles healthy. The stronger the muscles and tissues around your joints, the better able they are to support and protect those joints, even those that are weak and damaged from arthritis.

Your exercise program must be individualized depending on which joints are involved in your arthritis and the severity of involvement. If your arthritis is active, so that many joints are swollen, you will have to rest more and will not be able to do strengthening exercises. You should be able to do range-of-motion exercises, however. Ask your physician for guidance in this area.

Who can help me get started on an exercise program?

Your doctor can give you general advice about exercise and what exercises you should do. Physiatrists can help design and direct your exercise program. Physical therapists can show you special exercises to help keep your bones and muscles strong. Occupational therapists can show you how to perform activities in ways that will not place extra stress on your joints.

I'm a little afraid of exercising with arthritis. Are there risks?

Yes, there are some. A common risk is overworking your joints or muscles. This can happen if you exercise for too long or too hard, especially when you're just starting your exercise program. Your program must be designed especially for you and should take into account which joints are involved in your disease, your level of fitness, and the severity of your disease. By taking these precautions, you minimize the problems and increase the benefits. Ask your physician for more information on how to create a program tailored to meet your specific needs.

What kinds of exercise benefit people with arthritis?

People with arthritis benefit from a balanced exercise program that includes a variety of exercises. Three main types of exercises that should be included in your program are range-of-motion (flexibility), strengthening, and endurance exercises.

Range-of-Motion (Flexibility) Exercises

The range of motion (ROM) is the normal degree to which your joints can move in one direction or another. It is important to try to move your joints through their full range of motion every day. Daily activities such as housework, climbing stairs, dressing, cooking, lifting, and bending *do not* move your joints through their full range of motion. In other words, daily activities should not replace range-of-motion exercise. Even if your joints are painful and swollen, move them gently through their range of motion.

Strengthening Exercises

Strengthening exercises are beneficial because they help maintain and increase muscle strength. Strong muscles help keep your joints stable and more comfortable. Two common strengthening exercises for people with arthritis are isometric and isotonic exercises. It may be necessary to delay doing these exercises if the joints are inflamed and swollen.

- *Isometric exercises*—In these exercises, you tighten and help build your muscles without moving painful joints. Quadricep sets (tightening the large muscles at the front of your thighs) or gluteal sets (tightening the muscles in your buttocks) are examples of isometric exercises.
- *Isotonic exercises*—In these exercises, you move your joints to strengthen your muscles. Isotonic exercises seem like range-of-motion exercises, but they become strengthening exercises when you pick up the pace at which they are done or do them while holding light weights. You should add no more than one to two pounds initially. A good place to try isotonic exercises is in the water. In water, weight is not placed on weight-bearing joints and joint aggravation is therefore minimized.

HEALTH TIP

Try to move your joints through their full range of motion every day. Daily activities such as housework, climbing stairs, dressing, bathing, cooking, lifting or bending DO NOT move your joints through their full range of motion. Daily activities should NOT replace range-of-motion exercises.

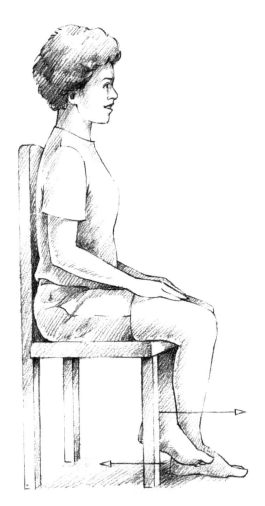

FIGURE 1
Isometric Exercise
This exercise strengthens the muscles that
bend and straighten your knee.
Sit in a straight-backed chair and cross
your ankles. Your legs can be almost
straight, or you can bend your knees
as much as you like. Push forward with
your back leg and press backward with
your front leg. Exert pressure evenly
so that your legs do not move. Hold and
count out loud for 10 seconds. Relax.
Change leg positions.

Strengthening exercises must be carefully designed for people with arthritis. Knowing which muscle needs to be strengthened and performing exercises without overstressing joints are key elements in a successful program. Your physical therapist, occupational therapist, and/or doctor can provide appropriate recommendations.

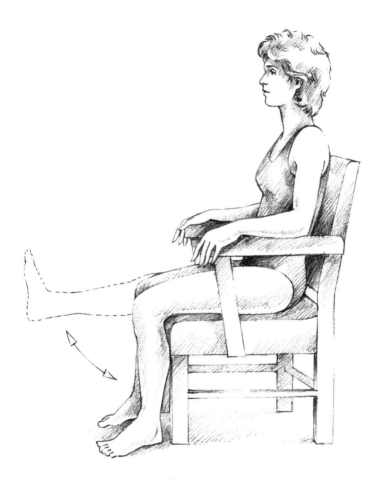

FIGURE 2
Isotonic Exercise
This exercise strengthens your thigh muscles. Sit in
a chair with both feet on the floor and spread slightly apart.
Raise one foot until your leg is as straight
as you can make it. Hold and count out loud for five
seconds. Gently lower your foot to the floor.
Relax. Repeat with your other leg.

79

Endurance Exercises

Endurance exercises are also good for people with arthritis because they strengthen the heart. They make your lungs more efficient and give you more stamina so you can work longer without tiring as quickly. Endurance exercises also help you sleep better, control your weight, and lift your spirits. Some of the most beneficial endurance exercises for people with arthritis are walking, exercising in water, and riding a stationary bicycle.

- *Walking*—Walking is an ideal exercise for people with arthritis because it puts less stress on joints than running, it requires no special skills, and it is inexpensive. The only equipment you will need is a good pair of walking shoes. Walking can be done at almost any time and anywhere. Many communities have walking or mall-walking clubs that provide both companionship and motivation. If you have severe hip, knee, ankle, or foot problems, though, talk with your doctor—walking may not be the right exercise for you.
- *Exercising in Water*—Swimming and exercise in warm water are especially good for stiff, sore joints because water helps support the body so there is less stress on your hips, knees, feet, and spine. Warm water also helps relax your muscles and decrease pain. The water should be between 83 and 90 degrees. You can do warm-water exercises while standing in shoulder- or chest-high

HEALTH TIP

Gradually build up your endurance exercises to 20 to 30 minutes per day, at least three times per week. Endurance exercises should be only one part of your total exercise program. DO NOT substitute endurance exercises for the therapeutic exercises your health-care team recommends.

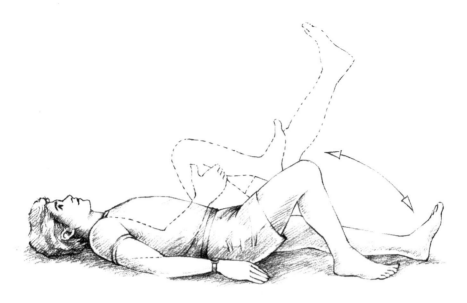

FIGURE 3

Knee and Hip

Lie on your back with one knee bent and the
other as straight as possible. Bend the knee of the
straight leg. Use your hands to pull your knee to
your chest. Push the leg into the air and then lower
it to the floor. Repeat, using the other leg. If you
feel pain in your knee, do not kick it into the
air. Just lower it to the floor.

water, or even while sitting down in shallow water. If you will be exercising in deeper water, bring along an inflatable tube or a floatation vest or belt to help keep you afloat.

• *Bicycling*—Bicycling, especially on an indoor stationary bicycle, is a good way to improve your fitness without putting too much stress on your hips, knees, and ankles. Adjust the seat height so that your knee straightens when the pedal is at its lowest point. Add resistance only after you have warmed up for five to ten minutes and only if it does not aggravate the joints, especially the hips, knees, and ankles. Exercise on a stationary bike should be started slowly, using limited or no resistance, particularly if you have knee problems.

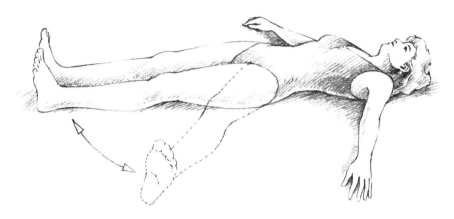

FIGURE 4

Hip

(Note: This exercise is not recommended for people who
have had total hip replacements, who have low back
problems or who have osteoporosis.) Lie on your back
with your legs straight and about six inches apart. Point
your toes up. Slide one leg out to the side and return.
Try to keep your toes pointing up. Slide your leg only.
Do not lift it. Repeat with your other leg. (This exercise
also can be done from a standing position.)

How can I get the greatest benefits from exercise?

Try exercising at different times of the day until you discover the time of
day that works best for you. Some people find that doing range-of-motion
exercises in the morning helps them loosen up for the day's activities; others
find that when they do gentle ROM exercises before going to bed, they're less
stiff in the morning. You may be most comfortable doing a few short sessions
of ROM exercises during different times of the day. As a general guideline,
exercise during the time of the day when you feel less pain and stiffness and
when you have enough time to do it properly.

Most important, exercise on a regular basis. Try to do your ROM exercises every day and your strengthening and endurance exercises every other day,
being careful not to aggravate swollen joints. Try to stay motivated even if
you miss a day; pick up again where you left off. If you miss several days,
though, you may need to begin exercising again at a lower level. Don't do
strenuous exercises just after eating or just before going to bed. And, finally,
wait at least two hours after a meal before exercising.

I've heard that warming up before exercising is important. Is this true?

Taking the time to warm up before exercising will help prevent injuries. Do gentle ROM and strengthening exercises for at least five to 10 minutes before you do more vigorous endurance-type exercise. Start your activity at a slow pace and gradually work up to a faster pace.

Using heat treatments or massage therapy before exercising is another effective way to warm up. Massage the stiff or sore areas or apply heat treatments to the area you will be exercising. Heat relaxes your joints and muscles and helps relieve pain. Cold also reduces pain for some people.

For more information on the correct use of heat or cold, see page 52.

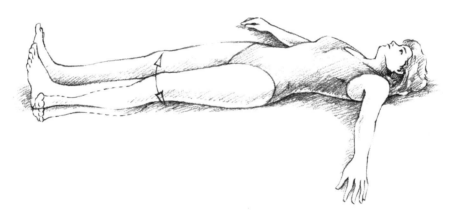

FIGURE 5
Hip and Knee
Lie on your back with your legs as straight as possible, about six inches apart. Keep your toes pointed up. Roll your hips and knees in and out, keeping your knees straight. To further strengthen knees, while lying with both legs out straight, attempt to push one knee down against the floor. Tighten the muscle on the front of the thigh. Hold this tightening for a slow count of five. Relax. Repeat with the other knee.

What are some other tips I should keep in mind while I'm exercising?

- *Don't hurry.* Initially, exercise at a comfortable, steady pace that allows you to speak without gasping for breath. Exercising at this pace gives your muscles time to relax between repetitions. With range-of-motion and flexibility exercises, it is better to do each exercise slowly and completely than to do a lot of repetitions at a fast pace. You can gradually increase the number of repetitions as you get into shape.

- *Remember to breathe while you exercise.* Don't hold your breath! Breathe out as you do the exercise, and breathe in as you relax between repetitions. Counting out loud during the exercise will help you concentrate on breathing deeply and regularly.

- *Watch for "warning signs" that you are exercising too hard.* Stop exercising right away if you feel tightness in your chest or experience severe shortness of breath or if you feel dizzy, faint, or sick to your stomach. If these symptoms occur, contact your doctor immediately. If you develop more joint pain or swelling, muscle pain, or a cramp, stop exercising and contact your

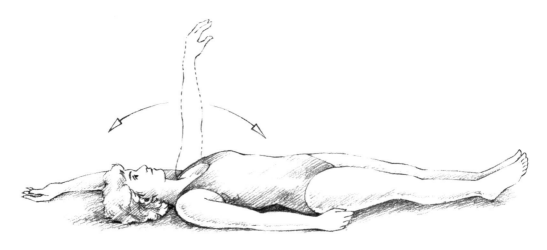

FIGURE 6
Shoulder
Lie on your back. Raise one arm over your head, keeping your elbow straight. Keep your arm close to your ear. Return your arm slowly to your side. Repeat with your other arm. (This exercise also can be done from a standing position.)

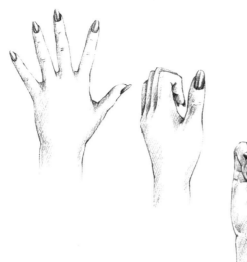
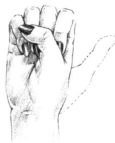

FIGURE 7

Fingers

Open your hand, with fingers straight and spread apart.
Bend all the finger joints except the knuckles. Touch the
top of your palm with your fingertips. Reach your thumb
across your palm until it touches the second joint of
your little finger. Stretch your thumb out and repeat.

EXERCISE TIPS

- Start with just a few exercises and slowly add more.

- "Listen" to your body. If it is telling you that your exercise hurts too
  much or is causing too much pain, stop. Ask your doctor to help you
  distinguish between normal exercise discomfort and the pain associated with too much exercise.

- If you have a flare (a period during which disease symptoms return
  or become worse), do only gentle range-of-motion exercises and
  talk to your doctor.

- Ask your local Arthritis Foundation chapter about joining a super-
  vised warm-water or land-exercise program. Many people find that
  exercising with a group is fun as well as healthy.

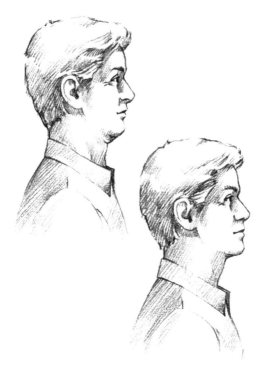

FIGURE 8
Chin and Neck
Pull your chin back as if to make a double
chin. Keep your head straight—don't look
down. Hold for three seconds. Then raise
your neck straight up as if someone were
pulling straight up on your hair.

physician for advice. You may need to change positions or the way you are
doing the exercise.

• *Know your body's signals.* During the first few weeks of your exercise
program, you may notice that your heart beats faster, you breathe faster,
and your muscles feel tense when you exercise. You may feel more tired at
night. These are normal reactions to exercise that indicate your body is
adapting to your new activities and getting into shape. These reactions
should become less noticeable each day.

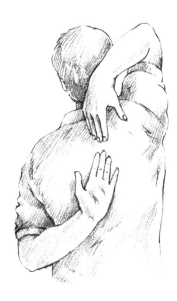

FIGURE 9

Back

Reach one palm over your shoulder
to pat your back and place the back
of your other hand on your lower
back. Slide hands toward each other,
trying to touch fingertips. (Note:
Many people are not able to actually
touch their fingertips together.)
Alternate arms.

THE TALK TEST

When you are exercising, you should be
able to talk easily and not be out of breath.
If you are exercising so hard that you can't
talk normally, you may need to slow down.

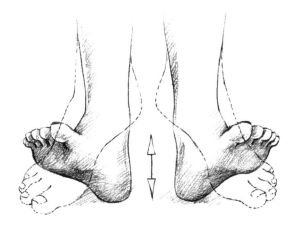

FIGURE 10
Ankle
While sitting, lift your toes as high as possible.
Then return your toes to the floor and lift
your heels as high as possible. Repeat.

• *Don't do too much too fast.* Building up your endurance should be a gradual process spread out over several weeks. Resist the temptation to do everything at once! You'll know you've done too much if you have joint or muscle pain that continues for two hours after exercising, or if your pain or fatigue is worse the next day. Next time, decrease the number of times you do each exercise and do the exercises more gently. If this doesn't help, ask your doctor or therapist about changing the exercise. If you experience more pain than usual, you need to stop and assess the situation. Pain is your most important warning sign that something is wrong.

Is it really important to cool down after exercising?

Yes, it is. After exercising, cool down for five to 10 minutes. This helps to slow down your heart, relax your muscles, and cool off your body. Cooling down is simply a matter of performing your exercises at a slower pace. Be sure to incorporate gentle stretching into your cool-down routine to avoid having stiff or sore muscles the next day.

I'm not sure I'll be able to stick to an exercise program. What will help me to keep going?

It's understandable that if you're in pain, you may feel depressed, and if you're depressed, you may not feel like moving or exercising. Keeping a positive attitude about yourself and your exercise program is important in keeping you motivated. One way to do this is to visualize daily the big picture of the long-term benefits of a regular exercise program. Think about how exercise can improve your quality of life. Exercise is a proven method for reducing pain and it helps you maintain stamina so you can keep up with most of your daily activities. Scale back on your exercise program on days when you don't feel like doing as much, but continue to do some type of exercise nonetheless.

The following tips may help you keep up with your program:

- Make exercise a regular part of your day
- Stay in the habit of doing at least some exercise even on those days when you aren't motivated
- Make an effort, because interrupting your routine can decrease the overall benefits you get from exercise
- Listen to your body's signals so you'll know when you need to either cut back or modify your program.

Exercise keeps your bones and muscles strong and your joints healthy, and it gives you more energy to keep up with daily activities. This is important for people with arthritis because exercise, when done properly, can decrease symptoms.

9

Diet and Arthritis

Can what we eat cause, cure, or affect arthritis? Because symptoms of arthritis can vary from day to day, it's natural to think that what you ate yesterday may have caused or reduced the pain you feel today.

Researchers are looking with increased interest at the role diet may play in arthritis. There are some scientific reasons to think certain foods might affect certain kinds of arthritis. In gout, for example, a definite dietary link exists.

This chapter answers questions you might have about your diet and provides information about various diet options that can lead to better health through proper nutrition.

Can the things I eat affect my arthritis?

Although scientists have not yet determined definitively whether what you eat affects the symptoms of your arthritis, they do know that a generally healthful diet can help you feel better overall. Variety, balance, and moderation are the keys to a healthful diet. A good diet includes some choices from each of the five food groups—grains, fruits, vegetables, dairy products, and meats—but the emphasis should be on grains, fruits, and vegetables. Eating a variety of foods gives you the 40 or more nutrients your body needs.

The pain, fatigue and depression of arthritis may decrease your appetite and make you disinterested in eating the variety of foods you need. And when you're feeling bad, cooking can seem like just another chore. Health professionals can help you learn more efficient cooking methods, so you'll be able to make a variety of easy-to-prepare yet healthy meals, even when you're feeling bad. Your doctor can refer you to an occupational therapist for advice on making cooking easier.

GUIDELINES FOR A HEALTHFUL DIET

- Eat a variety of foods.
- Maintain a healthy weight.
- Use fat and cholesterol in moderation.
- Eat plenty of vegetables, fruits and grain products.
- Use sugar in moderation.
- Use salt in moderation.
- Drink alcohol in moderation.
- Drink eight glasses of water a day.

How does diet affect gout?

Gout is the most familiar example of an arthritis-related disease in which there is a known link between the disease and diet. People with gout may have a painful attack if they eat foods with high levels of chemicals called purines. Animal meats are very rich in purines.

Purines are broken down into uric acid in the body. When you have gout, your body makes too much uric acid or has trouble getting rid of it. A buildup of uric acid can cause the symptoms of gout. Too much alcohol in the body can also interfere with the kidneys' ability to get rid of uric acid. Fortunately, medications are available that reduce excess uric acid. If you're taking gout medication, you may not have to change your diet. Your doctor may suggest, however, that you drink more fluids or monitor the intake of certain foods high in purines to help lower your uric acid level. (See Chapter 2 for more about gout.)

What is the connection between calcium and vitamins and osteoporosis?

Diets low in calcium or vitamin D may increase your chances of developing osteoporosis, a condition in which bones become thin and break easily (see Chapter 2 for more about osteoporosis.) Both calcium and vitamin D affect the strength of your bones.

Calcium is one of the main building blocks of bone. During the first thirty or so years of life, your bones are building up peak strength; then your bone mass levels off and eventually it decreases. To develop strong bones and then to prevent bone loss, most adults need to get 1,000 to 1,500 mg of calcium per day (more for teens, pregnant, or breast-feeding women or older adults).

Getting enough vitamin D is also important, because it increases the amount of calcium your body absorbs from your intestines. Vitamin D is produced by your body in response to sunlight. Good dietary sources of the vitamin include liver, fish oil, and fortified dairy products. Older people are especially prone to low vitamin D levels because they may not get out in the sun enough to meet their needs and their diets may be lacking in sufficient amounts of vitamins. You need 400 IU (international units) of vitamin D per day.

Is being overweight affecting my osteoarthritis?

People who are overweight have a higher risk of developing osteoarthritis and have more pain and disability if they get the disease. Being obese increases the risk of developing osteoarthritis in the weight-bearing joints such as knees, and possibly in the hips. People who are overweight tend to get osteoarthritis in the knees earlier in life, as opposed to those who are the ideal weight for their height.

If you're already overweight, the best thing to do is try to lose some weight. Even a few pounds can make a difference. Middle-aged women of average height who lose 10 pounds or more reduce their risk of knee osteoarthritis.

Can allergic reactions to foods affect my arthritis symptoms?

In rare cases, the body's immune system may react to certain foods in ways that may lead to or worsen the symptoms of some kinds of arthritis. Researchers suspect that in a small number of otherwise healthy people, symptoms of arthritis have developed as a result of an allergic reaction to food. For most people who have thought that their arthritis symptoms were related to food, a connection between food and those symptoms could not be confirmed.

Is losing weight by fasting or going on low-calorie/low-fat diets harmful if I have arthritis?

Researchers have observed that fasting and low-calorie/low-fat/low-protein diets slightly reduce some of the symptoms of rheumatoid arthritis in humans or of lupus in animals. This is because the active immune response in diseases such as rheumatoid arthritis is inhibited during fasting. But because fasting can cause you to lose muscle and can produce other harmful effects, it isn't recommended as a treatment for arthritis. Because people with inflammatory diseases such as rheumatoid arthritis have been shown to have low muscle mass, fasting may be especially harmful to them.

A vegetarian diet may be helpful in modifying disease activity in people with rheumatoid arthritis. Eating foods in the lower levels of the Food Pyramid, which are the basis of a healthful diet for anyone, provides them with all the nutrients they need.

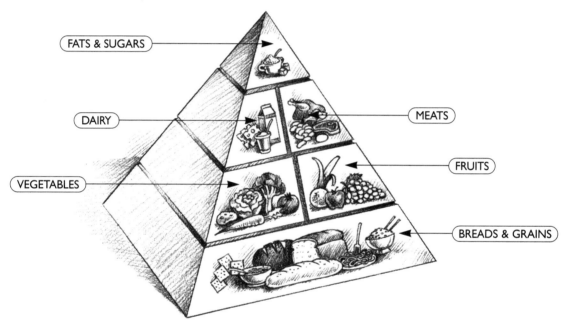

Following the Food Guide Pyramid can help you eat a well-balanced diet that consists primarily of grains, fruits, and vegetables.

Credit: U.S. Department of Agriculture/U.S. Department of Health and Human Services.

What role do fatty acids play in improving arthritis symptoms?

Certain fatty acids are known to play a role in chemical changes in the body, but exactly what that role is and how those changes affect arthritis inflammation is still being studied. For instance, oils from some cold-water fish (salmon, mackerel, and herring, for example) block the body from making some of the substances that cause painful inflammation in people with rheumatoid arthritis. Studies have shown that people with rheumatoid arthritis have had modest improvement in their pain from tender joints after taking large amounts of fatty acids (called omega-3 fatty acids) from fish oils over a period of time. However, it is difficult and sometimes not palatable to take the quantity of omega-3 fatty acids taken daily during the study. A compromise would be to have two meals of cold-water fish each week and ideally more frequently. Supplementation with omega-3 fatty acids should be done only under your doctor's supervision.

What is a good diet?

Experts in diet have formulated basic guidelines for a balanced, healthful diet. Eat a variety of foods; maintain a healthy weight; use fat and cholesterol in moderation; eat plenty of vegetables, fruits, and grain products; use sugar in moderation; use salt (sodium chloride) in moderation; drink alcohol in moderation, and drink eight glasses of water a day.

Can my arthritis medications affect how my body processes food?

Certain kinds of medications can affect how well your body uses what you eat. For example, corticosteroids cause your body to lose potassium, retain sodium, and gain weight. Some antacids, which may be taken to reduce stomach irritation, also contain high levels of sodium, calcium, and magnesium. It's important to know this if you have kidney problems, which can make it harder for your body to regulate these important minerals.

Most people who eat a variety of foods maintain adequate levels of nutrients. Talk with your doctor about how the medications you are taking can affect your nutritional status and whether it might be useful to take a vitamin supplement.

I'd like to lose a little weight because my doctor said it might help ease some of my arthritis symptoms. What's the best way to do this?

Extra pounds put stress on your joints, which increases your risk of developing osteoarthritis in the knees and possibly in the hips, because these joints bear the weight of the body. If you already have knee osteoarthritis, it's important to control your weight. A registered dietitian and your doctor can

MAKE MEAL PREPARATION EASIER

- Plan rest breaks during meal preparation time.
- Use good posture while cooking.
- Keep the things you use most often out on the counter.
- Occasionally use convenience foods to reduce the strain of cooking meals.
- Add fresh fruit and bread to a frozen dinner to make a complete, satisfying meal.
- Purchase pre-sliced and -chopped vegetables from the produce or frozen food sections of grocery stores.
- Use kitchen gadgets and appliances such as electric can openers and microwave ovens to make cooking tasks easier.

help you work out a lifelong weight management plan that is right for you.

A good weight management plan will include balance, variety, and moderation in your diet, as well as regular exercise. Cutting down on foods high in fat and sugar can be tough, but the health benefits are well worth the effort. Achieving a healthy body weight will help reduce the progression of osteoarthritis—not to mention that you'll look and feel better. A daily walk or swim is a good way to exercise without having to place undue stress on joints that are already stressed by extra weight.

Are there any tried-and-true food preparation tips if I'm trying to lose weight?

Avoid food high in fat and cholesterol. Many adults with arthritis also have high blood pressure or heart disease. Reducing the fat and cholesterol in your diet will be helpful for these conditions as well. Fat is a source of concentrated calories. Choose low-fat cuts of meat and low-fat dairy products, and limit how much fat you add to your diet by avoiding high-fat salad dressings and nuts and nut butters. A daily serving of meat or fish the size of one deck of playing cards (i.e., a serving size of 3 ounces) is adequate for most adults. Egg yolks should be limited to three per week. The challenge of cooking and preparing food with less oil is getting easier, as food manufacturers become aware of the benefits of reducing fat. New products, recipes, and preparation methods are becoming available almost daily.

What foods are good to eat?

Eat plenty of vegetables, fruits, and grain products. Fruits, vegetables, and whole-grain products help give you energy and keep your bowels regular. Most of these foods are also low in fat, high in fiber and are important sources of vitamins and nutrients. If you include plenty of variety in your diet, by sampling different kinds of fruits and vegetables, you will probably develop a taste for these more healthful foods. Foods high in complex carbohydrates (e.g., breads, pasta, potatoes) are useful in weight control if used in moderate quantities and they help meet your body's energy needs. Avoid adding heavy sauces and gravies, however, because these can be high in sodium and fat.

Whole-grain products (e.g., whole wheat breads, cereals) are also excellent sources of fiber. Fiber comes from the parts of plants that your body can't digest. Some types of fibers help soften stools and contribute to more rapid elimination of wastes, thus preventing constipation.

What items could "sabotage" my diet?

Sugar, salt (sodium), and alcohol need to be used in moderation. Sugar makes food sweet, but it also adds calories and promotes weight gain. When you're at the grocery store checking food packages for the sugar content in foods, look for words such as *dextrose, sucrose, fructose, honey* and *dextrin* to determine whether sugar has been added.

Salt (sodium) causes the body to retain water, which can affect blood pressure. Fast foods and processed foods may be convenient, but often they contain large amounts of sodium. In addition, some arthritis drugs, such as corticosteroids, may cause the body to retain too much sodium. Now's the time to find out if your favorite restaurant offers low-salt or no-salt food choices. And be a smart consumer when you do your grocery shopping by reading labels to find out how much salt is added to the foods you enjoy. Ask your grocer about low-salt or no-salt alternatives. Your doctor or dietitian can also talk to you about whether it would be helpful to use a salt substitute.

Can I drink alcohol if I have arthritis?

Alcohol can have many adverse effects on your health and should be avoided if you are taking certain arthritis medications. For instance, stomach irritation and bleeding are more likely to occur if you drink alcohol while you are taking aspirin or other NSAIDs. And too much alcohol combined with too much acetaminophen can damage the liver.

In addition, alcohol can increase the amount of uric acid in the blood and aggravate gout. Methotrexate combined with alcohol can also cause liver damage. Talk with your doctor about drinking, even in moderation, while you are taking arthritis medication. Alcohol can also add unwanted pounds, because it adds extra calories to your diet.

What should I be looking for on food labels?

Beginning in 1994, new nutrition labels were required for most foods. Many packages already listed ingredients, but there were no standards for

Nutrition Facts

Serving Size 1 cup (30g)
Servings Per Container 12

Amount Per Serving

Calories 90	Calories from Fat 10

	% Daily Value*
Total Fat 1g	**2**%
Saturated Fat 0g	**0**%
Cholesterol 0mg	**0**%
Sodium 190mg	**8**%
Total Carbohydrate 22g	**7**%
Dietary Fiber 3g	**12**%
Sugars 9g	
Protein 3g	

Vitamin A	25%	•	Vitamin C	0%
Calcium	0%	•	Iron	25%

* Percent Daily Values are based on a 2,000 calorie diet. Your daily values may be higher or lower depending on your calorie needs:

	Calories	2,000	2,500
Total Fat	Less than	65g	80g
Sat Fat	Less than	20g	25g
Cholesterol	Less than	300mg	300mg
Sodium	Less than	2,400mg	2,400mg
Total Carbohydrate		300g	375g
Fiber		25g	30g

Calories per gram:
Fat 9 • Carbohydrate 4 • Protein 4

American Heart Association

New food labels make
it easy to compare
food choices so you know
what you're eating.

comparing one food with another. The new labeling allows you to read the nutritional content of the foods so you can make smarter choices for a more healthful diet. The Food Labeling Act also set new guidelines for the health claims food manufacturers can make. Claims such as "fat free," "cholesterol free," "low sodium" and others are now defined by government standards.

Remembering these key words will help you judge nutritional content: *free* means the product has the least amount of that nutrient; *very low* and *low* means the product has a little more; and *reduced* or *less* means the food has 25 percent less of that nutrient than the standard version of the food.

Is one eating plan better for people with arthritis than another?

There is not yet enough scientific evidence to tell if one diet is better for people with arthritis than another. For this reason, any claims that a special diet improves arthritis symptoms are unproven. However, researchers emphasize the importance of eating a healthful diet if you have arthritis. There are three ways you can improve your diet and get on track toward healthful eating:

1. Add variety to your diet and eat more foods high in fiber and complex carbohydrates.

2. Reduce your intake of salt, fat, cholesterol, sugar, and alcohol.

3. Take in the daily requirements of minerals and vitamins (especially calcium and vitamin D).

Such changes are easier to say than to make, but making these changes will certainly help you to achieve and maintain a healthy weight—the foundation for improved quality of life for many people with arthritis.

1 0

Joint Protection

As many people learn the hard way, overusing joints affected by arthritis can make the pain worse. There are ways to reduce the stress to your joints during daily activities, but it may take a while before these joint-protection techniques seem natural to you. Learning to recognize when you feel healthy enough to do certain tasks and when you should avoid putting excess stress on joints is important in managing your pain and fatigue. This chapter answers questions about joint protection and describes a number of ways to improve your posture and body mechanics.

What is joint protection?

Joint protection involves doing certain tasks differently to avoid putting excess stress on joints. Three methods are commonly used to make daily tasks easier:

- *Joint positioning*—Using your joints more efficiently reduces the amount of stress you put on them. Use your larger or stronger joints to pick up bags, boxes, or heavy objects and spread the load over stronger joints or larger areas of your body. By bending slightly at the knees before picking up large items, for example, you can absorb most of the weight in the quadricep (thigh) muscles in your legs as opposed to the muscles in your back. Also try to use your forearms and the palms of your hands instead of your fingers when you need to carry things.
- *Using assistive devices*—Canes, crutches, or walkers may help you put less stress on the joints that carry your full body weight. Utensils with larger handles, pens with built-up grips, and reachers are other devices that can ease joint stress.

• *Controlling weight*—It really helps to maintain your recommended weight or to try and lose weight in order to reduce the risk of developing osteoarthritis in the knees. If you already have osteoarthritis in the knees, losing weight can help reduce stress on your knee joints and may lessen the pain. Talk to your doctor about other ways to protect your joints.

What does "distributing my load" mean?

Distributing your load, or spreading around your weight to as many major muscle groups as possible when you need to, is another way to reduce excess stress on any one joint. For example, carry your purse or golf bag with a shoulder strap rather than in your hand. This protects elbow, wrist, or finger joints and also keeps your back muscles in better alignment. When you climb stairs, try to use your stronger leg first. Conversely, when you go down stairs, use your weaker leg first.

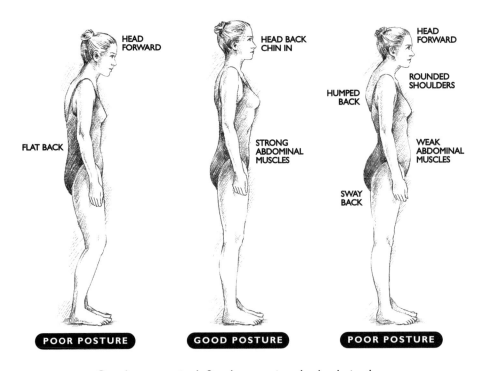

Good posture is defined as putting the body in the most efficient and least stressful position. Bad posture is more tiring and adds to your pain.

How do self-help devices work?

Self-help devices take stress off joints and can make tasks easier and more efficient, especially when you're tired, stiff, or in a hurry. These products can provide leverage to give you more force (e.g., lever faucet and tap turners, aids with lever handles to open push-button car doors); keep joints and muscles in the best position for function (i.e., a pizza cutter, instead of a knife); extend your reach if your range of motion is limited (e.g., long-handled shoehorns, reachers, and bath brushes); and help you avoid strain on joints and muscles altogether (e.g., electric can openers, toothbrushes, meat slicers, grooming aids). Using self-help products requires less energy and can relieve stress on your muscles and joints.

Sometimes I know that I need help because of my arthritis pain, but I'm hesitant to ask. How should I handle this?

Although it may be hard to admit that some things are more difficult to do than before, it's important to get help when you need it. This is especially true of activities that place a lot of stress on your joints and that may cause pain and/or fatigue. Your family and friends will understand you and your condition better if you share your feelings with them and let them know how they can help.

11

Surgery

Most people with arthritis will never need surgery. Their arthritis can be managed with nonsurgical treatment—medication, exercise, physical and occupational therapy, rest, and joint protection. If you have significant pain and joint damage, however, surgery could provide relief from the pain and better range of motion.

Your doctor and a surgeon will determine if joint surgery might help you. The decision to have surgery is a major one. It isn't a decision to be made quickly and without good reasons. You need to be fully informed about what will happen if you decide to go forward with surgery, and you need to know about alternative options if you decide against it. Your doctor should tell you as much as possible about what to expect.

This chapter addresses the most common questions about arthritis surgery, including the benefits, the types of procedures that are available (i.e., synovectomy, osteotomy, arthrodesis/bone fusion, arthroplasty, total joint replacement, and arthroscopy), the risks involved, the value of a second opinion, and the cost, as well as questions you might want to ask your doctor before surgery.

When will my physician suggest or recommend joint surgery?

Some people with arthritis have constant pain that interferes with their activities and sometimes with their sleep. Your physician will suggest surgery when you have significant joint damage resulting in this level of pain. Relief of pain is the most important benefit of joint surgery.

Your surgeon will discuss the reason he or she is recommending surgery, the type of surgery that is being considered, what to expect during recovery,

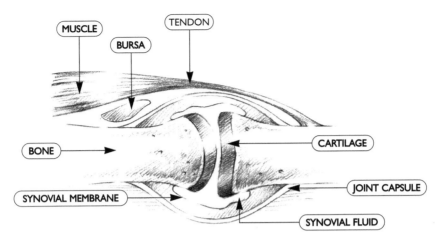

MUSCLE
BURSA
TENDON
BONE
CARTILAGE
SYNOVIAL MEMBRANE
JOINT CAPSULE
SYNOVIAL FLUID

**Understanding the structure of
your joints helps you understand
what surgery can do for you.**

and the results that you should expect. You must make sure that the results you expect can be achieved with the surgery. You may want the surgery to result in complete restoration of the motion of a joint, for example, whereas your surgeon may inform you that the surgery will control the pain but you will still have limited motion. You must understand what the surgery will accomplish and what it won't accomplish. Even if your doctor thinks that surgery can help you, there are still many things you need to know before making a final decision.

What are some of the benefits of surgery?

Joint surgery can offer several benefits. Relief of pain is usually the major benefit if the joint has been damaged. Many people with arthritis are in constant pain. Some of this pain can be relieved by rest, heat and cold treatments, exercise, splints, and medication. When these therapies don't help, surgery may be considered.

Improved movement and use of a joint are other important benefits of joint surgery. Continuous inflammation and the wearing away of bone and cartilage can cause joints, tendons, and ligaments to become damaged or pulled out of place. Losing the use of a joint can hamper your activities. When this happens, surgery to replace or stabilize the joint may be suggested. An improvement in the alignment of deformed joints, especially in the hand, can be expected with some types of surgery.

What are some of the risks of surgery?

If you have serious problems with your lungs or heart, the risks of anesthesia and surgery may be too great for you. Before any kind of surgery, it's important to have other health problems evaluated and under control. For example, any type of bacterial infection must be cleared up before surgery, so you do not risk infecting the new joint. Another potential problem after surgery is the development of blood clots in the legs. This risk can be decreased by using blood-thinning drugs. Being overweight puts extra stress on the heart and lungs. If you're overweight, recovery of the use of a weight-bearing joint (hip or knee) may also be slower and the resulting joint function less than optimal. Discuss these and other potential problems with your regular arthritis doctor and with the surgeon.

What are some of the questions I should ask my surgeon before considering joint surgery?

There are many questions you should ask: What will happen during the operation? Do you have written materials or videotapes of this surgery that I can review? How long will the surgery take? Can it be performed on an outpatient basis? What risks are involved in the surgery, and how likely are they to occur? Are blood transfusions necessary, and, if so, can I donate my own blood? What type of anesthesia will I have, and what are the risks involved? How much improvement can I expect? Will additional surgery be necessary? If surgery is chosen, will you be in contact with my regular doctor and will he or she be involved while I am in the hospital? Are you board certified, and do you specialize in arthritis surgery? What is your experience with doing this kind of surgery? Must I stop any of my medications before surgery? What happens if I wait to have surgery? Are there any risks if I don't have surgery?

What questions should I ask beforehand about my post-surgery recovery?

Again, there are many questions you should ask: How long will I need to stay in the hospital? How much pain will I have, and will I receive medication for it? How long after surgery might my pain last? When will I begin physical therapy? Will I need home or outpatient therapy? Are physical therapy, occupational therapy, and home health care covered by insurance? (You may need to get this information from your insurance company.) Will I need to arrange for special help at home, and if so for how long? (Again, you may need to ask

SUGGESTED QUESTIONS TO ASK YOUR DOCTOR

IT MAY BE HARD TO REMEMBER WHAT YOU WANT TO ASK
YOUR DOCTOR. HERE ARE SOME QUESTIONS YOU MAY WANT
TO ASK AT YOUR NEXT APPOINTMENT.

ABOUT THE SURGERY

- What kinds of treatment may I consider other than surgery?
- How successful will these treatments be?
- Can you explain the operation?
- Do you have written materials or videotapes of this surgery
  that I can review?
- How long will the surgery take?
- Can it be performed on an outpatient basis?
- What risks are involved in the surgery? How likely are they?
- Are blood transfusions necessary? If so, can I donate my own blood?
- What type of anesthesia will I have? What are the risks?
- How much improvement can I expect?
- Will more surgery be necessary?
- If surgery is chosen, will my family doctor be involved
  in my hospital stay? In what way?
- Are you board-certified, and do you have a special interest
  in arthritis surgery?
- What is your experience doing this type of surgery?
- Is an exercise program recommended before and after the operation?
- Must I stop any of my medications before surgery?
- What happens if I delay surgery?
- What are the risks if I don't have surgery?

AFTER SURGERY

- How long will I stay in the hospital?
- What pain is normal to expect? How long will it last? Will I
  receive any type of medication for it?
- How long do I have to stay in bed?
- When do I start physical therapy? Will I need home or outpatient therapy?
- Are physical therapy, occupational therapy and home health care covered by
  insurance? (You may need to address this question to your insurance company.)
- Will I need to arrange for special help at home? If so, for how long? Is
  it covered by my insurance?
- What medications will I need at home, and how long will I need to take them?
- What limits will there be on my activities — driving, climbing stairs, bending?
- How often will I have follow-up visits with you? Are these visits covered by
  insurance? Are they included in the cost of the surgery?

someone at your insurance company what is covered.) What medications will I need at home and how long will I need to take them? What limits will there be on my activities—driving, climbing stairs, bending? How often will I have follow-up visits with you? Are the visits covered by insurance, and are they included in the cost of the surgery? (You may need to check with your insurance company about this, too.)

Why is getting a second opinion a good idea?

If you're not sure about having surgery, seek a second opinion from another surgeon with arthritis surgery experience. Sign a release form and ask that your medical records and X-rays be sent to the consulting surgeon. Consider the advice of all your doctors carefully before making your decision.

I'm concerned about the cost of joint surgery. What should I expect?

The cost will vary depending on many factors: the rates charged by the surgeon, anesthesiologist, and hospital; the type of surgery being performed; the medications you will need; physical therapy requirements; types of implants used; whether special tests are required; and the length of your hospital stay. Check with your doctor, insurance company, and (if you qualify) Medicaid or Medicare to find out what your coverage includes. Do this *before* the surgery so you won't have any unpleasant surprises.

GETTING A SECOND OPINION

If you're not sure about having surgery, ask for a second opinion from another doctor. Ask your doctor to suggest a surgeon with arthritis experience. Sign a release form and ask that your medical records and X-rays be sent to the consulting physician. Consider the advice of all your doctors carefully.

u have already spent time in a hospital during the year, you should
ur insurance policy for benefits coverage during the remainder of the
,ou are in a managed care plan, your coverage may require a second
opinion before surgery and may also specify the number of days that you may
spend in the hospital before and after surgery.

What kinds of surgery are available?

• *Synovectomy*—This procedure removes diseased synovium (joint lining)
in a single joint or several adjacent joints. The removal of the diseased
synovium reduces the pain and swelling of rheumatoid arthritis, for example, and may prevent or slow down damage to that joint.

• *Osteotomy*—This procedure corrects bone deformity by cutting and
repositioning deformed bone. Osteotomy of the tibia (shin bone) is occasionally performed to correct curvature and the weight-bearing position of
the lower leg in people with osteoarthritis of the knee.

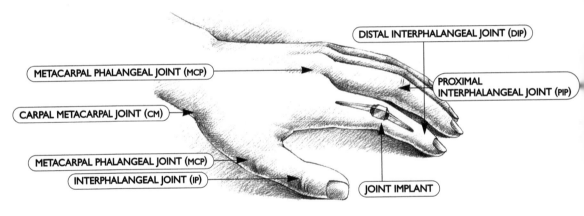

DISTAL INTERPHALANGEAL JOINT (DIP)

METACARPAL PHALANGEAL JOINT (MCP)

PROXIMAL INTERPHALANGEAL JOINT (PIP)

CARPAL METACARPAL JOINT (CM)

METACARPAL PHALANGEAL JOINT (MCP)

INTERPHALANGEAL JOINT (IP)

JOINT IMPLANT

THE HAND

In each finger, three areas can be affected by arthritis. The most common are the knuckle (MCP) and
middle (PIP) joints, which are more likely to be
replaced with implants. The joint closest to the tip
of the finger (DIP) may be fused if it causes a problem. Both the base of the thumb (MCP) and the
joint closest to the tip of the thumb (IP) can be
fused or replaced with an implant.

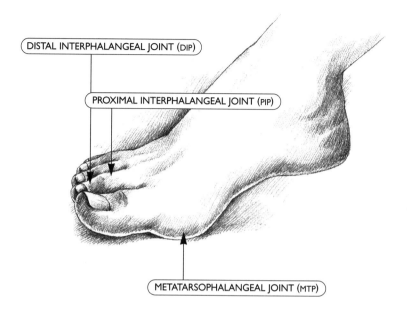

DISTAL INTERPHALANGEAL JOINT (DIP)

PROXIMAL INTERPHALANGEAL JOINT (PIP)

METATARSOPHALANGEAL JOINT (MTP)

THE FOOT

Surgery on joints of the foot is most often used to treat the painful and disfiguring effects of arthritis. If arthritis affects the joints of the great toe, the base of the great toe (MTP) or the joint closest to the end of the toe (DIP) may be fused, removed, and in rare instances, replaced with an implant.

• *Resection*—During this procedure, part or all of a bone is removed. It is often done when diseased joints in the foot make walking very painful and difficult. Resection is also done to remove painful bunions. Resection on part of the wrist or elbow can help improve function and relieve pain.

• *Arthrodesis/bone fusion*—In this surgery, the two bones forming a joint are fused together permanently. This enables the fused joint to bear weight better and become more stable and therefore less painful. The procedure is usually done to relieve pain in the ankles, wrists, thumbs, and big toe.

• *Arthroplasty*—This surgery involves the rebuilding of joints. Joints may be resurfaced and relined or totally replaced.

- *Total joint replacement*—In a joint replacement, surgeons remove a diseased joint and replace it with an artificial implant made of a flexible material. Total joint replacement has been widely used for many years and the results are excellent, especially with hips and knees. Other joints, such as the shoulders, elbows, and knuckles, may also be replaced.
- *Arthroscopy*—In this procedure, a tiny instrument called an arthroscope is inserted into the joint, which enables the doctor to look at the joint and possibly remove tissue. Arthroscopic surgery can be used to find out what kind of arthritis exists and how much damage is present. People usually recover from arthroscopic surgery more quickly than if the joint is surgically opened.

What can I do to prepare myself for surgery?

Preparing mentally and physically for surgery is an important step toward a successful result. If you are knowledgeable about the process, you are more likely to have a swifter recovery and fewer problems.

If you smoke, you're going to need to stop before surgery. A well-balanced diet is important to your overall health, but it is especially important around the time of surgery. You might want to take multi-vitamins if you feel your diet is insufficient.

Because aspirin and NSAIDs can interfere with blood clotting, you must stop taking them before surgery. If you take cortisone, Prednisone, or any other steroid medication, you must tell your surgeon before the operation. Not only should these medications not be stopped before or after surgery, but your doctor is likely to want to increase your dosage at the time of surgery. Tell your doctor what drugs you are taking and he or she will advise you on which medications to take before and after your operation.

What can I expect after surgery?

Depending on the type of surgery you have, your doctor will usually prescribe rest, physical therapy, and limited activity. You may need days or weeks of rest. In addition, you may need to use splints, a cane, a walker, a wheelchair, or crutches before you are able to perform your usual tasks. Talk with your doctor about any short-term limitations you can expect and anything else to expect during the recovery period. You may also be referred to an occupational therapist for advice on how to do daily activities in ways that put the least stress on your joints.

As soon as you're able, and depending on the type of surgery you've had, you will begin physical therapy.

What can I expect during physical therapy?

Be prepared to work hard. If you don't, your repaired joint may be less useful than it could be. Some pain is common during the early stages of physical therapy. This pain usually comes from the muscles, not the joint. Some of your muscles may not have been used much or may have been working in abnormal ways to protect a sore joint.

It's important to understand that muscles get stronger in response to exercise. An exercise that hurts today may hurt a little less tomorrow. You will see improvements in range of motion, along with decreased pain, as you go through your therapy. It is very important to be dedicated to your physical therapy. Results take time, but the rewards can be great. If you have questions about pain or lack of progress, talk with your therapist and surgeon.

What if I still have some reservations about surgery?

Joint surgery is not for everyone. Even if your doctor and surgeon determine that surgery will improve your condition, the decision to have surgery is up to you. You should weigh each of your options and understand all that surgery will involve. Your commitment to surgery is a key ingredient to its success.

Of course, you will have support in this undertaking. A team of doctors, nurses, physical and occupational therapists, and social workers will work to make your surgery successful. Family and friends are also part of your team. Look to them for emotional support and for assistance during your recovery. But always keep in mind that the most important team member is you.

12

Unproven Remedies

Although many treatments have been proven to reduce the pain and loss of motion associated with arthritis, many other products are available whose effects are unproven. Unproven remedies are treatments that have not been shown to be effective and safe in controlled scientific tests. Some of these treatments are health frauds that have been promoted for profit by people who can offer no scientific basis for their claims. Other treatments are promising but are still under study. They, too, are considered unproven until they have been shown through studies and statistical tests to work and to be safe. Still other treatments are unproven because their effects and safety have not been studied at all.

Before you try a treatment for arthritis that is not prescribed by your doctor, it is important to answer these three questions: Is it likely to work for me? How safe is it? How is it promoted? This chapter will help answer these and other questions about unproven remedies.

I've heard about several alternative treatments for my arthritis from friends. Should I try one?

You often have to judge claims for unproven remedies for yourself. Some of these remedies are harmless. Some are harmful. Others have effects that are unknown. Any unproven remedy can hurt you if it delays appropriate treatment or if you abandon the medical treatment prescribed by your physician.

You should discuss any alternative treatment you are considering with your physician.

How can an unproven remedy hurt me?

Even an unproven remedy that is in itself harmless can be unsafe if it causes you to stop or slow down prescribed treatments that you are taking for your arthritis. Scientific studies of proven treatments for arthritis have shown that they are relatively safe and effective. To be "effective," a treatment must meet one or more of the following criteria: reduce pain, reduce inflammation, keep joints moving, and keep you independent.

Some unproven remedies, like copper bracelets, are ineffective but harmless. Other remedies can have a direct negative effect on your health. L-tryptophan, for example, was promoted in health food stores several years ago for insomnia and was used for treating fibromyalgia. It was shown to cause a disease called eosinophilia myalgia syndrome, a condition characterized by muscle aches, an increase in a type of white blood cells called eosinophilia, frequent swelling of the hands and feet, a rash, cough, and peripheral neuropathy (damage to the nerves in the arms and legs). A small percentage of those affected died from the disease.

SOME COMMON UNPROVEN REMEDIES FOR ARTHRITIS

HARMLESS
Copper bracelets
Mineral springs
Vibrators

HARMFUL
Dimethyl Sulphamethoxide (DMSO)
Large doses of vitamins
Topical snake venom
Injectable bee venom
Drugs with hidden ingredients,
such as steroids (Butazolidin)

UNKNOWN
Lasers
Yucca
Uranium mines

What are some other examples of unproven remedies?

Many of the special diets you may have read about for arthritis are unproven. As yet, their effects have not been studied. Most of the nutrients promoted in health food stores as helpful in reducing the symptoms of arthritis are also unproven. Remember, products sold in health food stores do not have to be proven to be effective or safe. Other unproven remedies are DMSO, snake venom, bee venom, large doses of vitamins, and mineral springs, to name a few. Some treatments are new or experimental, which means they are still being studied. An example of an experimental drug showing promise in controlled studies is cyclosporine, which is usually used to suppress the immune system in people who have had organ transplants. These studies are determining the effectiveness of cyclosporine in controlling arthritis and the risks of possible side effects.

Why would someone with arthritis try an unproven remedy?

When people with a chronic type of arthritis feel they have tried all the medical profession has to offer and hear from well-meaning people about unproven remedies with supposedly miraculous cures, they are often tempted to try them. These alleged cures are sold to all who ask for them—some of whom don't have arthritis, some of whom have mild forms, and some of whom have a type of arthritis in which the symptoms come and go. As a result, some people will feel better and attribute their improvement to the unproven remedy, when in fact the improvement had little to do with the remedy, except for the placebo effect. The placebo effect is the positive benefit people experience at least temporarily when they are given something that they believe will help them. As you can imagine, there will be some people who get better and their stories will be promoted. Were those people really like you? Did they have severe rheumatoid arthritis?

How can I avoid being "taken in" by someone promoting an unproven remedy?

Promoters of unproven remedies offer an answer for your problems with arthritis. Ads often make false or exaggerated claims that the remedy will cure the disease; it is natural and will produce no side effects; it will work for all types of arthritis; it will work for other ailments; using the remedy will require no effort on your part; it will be inexpensive; it will work immediately and permanently; or it will eliminate the need for drugs or surgery. Suspect health fraud when you see or hear these claims. If the claim seems too good to be true, be skeptical.

Are there ways I can spot an unproven remedy?

You can identify an unproven remedy by asking what's known about its effects, its ingredients, its safety, and how it is promoted. Often the only source of information on a remedy is what's given out by its promoters. If the product does not include details about the ingredients and potential side effects, be suspicious. Check with your doctor or local chapter of the Arthritis Foundation for more information before you try a remedy.

What if a study of a particular "remedy" has been conducted ?

A single study may get optimistic results, but in *repeated* studies the results may be different. A single study only suggests that a treatment has promise. To prove that a treatment really works, a number of scientists must repeat the study and get similar results.

This chart lists some common diets, supplements or remedies for which unproven claims have been made. For some, there are studies or case reports about the claim. The effects or safety of many other items on the list are unknown.

SOME UNPROVEN DIETS AND SUPPLEMENTS FOR ARTHRITIS

DIET/SUPPLEMENT

Alfalfa
Black walnuts
Copper
Copper salts
Glucosamine sulfate
Immune power diet
No meats/preservatives diet
No nightshades diet
Plant oils
Sodium nitrate
Vinegar and honey
Zinc

The study must also have had a control group. One group of people tries the new treatment. This is the experimental group. A second group gets a treatment whose effects are already known, or they get no treatment at all. This comparison group is known as the control group. Using control groups helps to show that the results of a study are due to the new treatment and not other factors, such as the placebo effect.

What if I'm told that the treatment will work for all types of arthritis?

Be skeptical. There are more than 100 types of arthritis, and proven treatments vary for each kind. If you hear about a treatment that works for arthritis, ask what kind of arthritis the people in the study had. Keep in mind that scientists test new treatments on people with a specific type of arthritis, and these people are similar to the control group in age, sex, race, medical history, and the features of their specific disease.

What about case histories and testimonials?

Again, be skeptical. Case histories or testimonials are stories about a treatment that worked for only a few people. They often use the person's name and picture. Scientists look for a treatment to show improvements in a large number of people in controlled and repeated studies and using statistical tests. Large numbers, controlled studies, and statistical tests show that the results are not due to chance or to the placebo effect. Scientists do not reveal the names of people involved in their studies except under special circumstances and with the patients' permission.

How will I know if a treatment is safe?

Suspect that a "remedy" may be unproven if it does not include directions or a list of the contents. There should be warnings on the label or instructions stating who should not use the treatment. Some side effects of unproven remedies can be very serious. You need to know beforehand how any new treatment is likely to affect you. Always consult with your doctor, who can help you weigh the benefits against any possible risks.

What if I'm told that a treatment is natural or harmless?

Many people think that natural means harmless. Scientists look for tests to prove that a treatment is safe and has some benefits. For example, snake venom is natural, but its effects can be harmful. Also, many natural substances can be harmful if taken in excessive amounts.

How do I know whether I should try some new arthritis medication?

Ask your doctor. As noted previously, you can often spot an unproven remedy by how and where it is promoted. Promoters of unproven remedies use many methods to appeal directly to people with arthritis, their families, and their friends. These methods include the media—television, radio news, talk shows, newspapers, and magazines. Again, your doctor can advise you about the reliability of alternative remedies.

Could these inventors of unproven remedies have a secret formula that will cure arthritis?

Scientists share their discoveries so that other experts in arthritis can review and validate the results and share in the benefits for patients. A claim that only its inventor knows about a new discovery is a signal that the remedy is unproven.

Claims of "curing" arthritis should also be suspect. Because there are many different kinds of arthritis, it's unlikely that one treatment will cure them all. If there's a major new advance in the treatment of arthritis, your physician will know about it.

Can I trust treatment claims made in the media?

Newspapers, magazines, television, and books are sometimes good sources of information about how to deal with arthritis, but they should not be your only point of reference. Research on new treatments will appear first in medical journals that are read by experts in arthritis care. If you have questions about a treatment you've seen or heard about, check with your doctor or local Arthritis Foundation chapter.

If I decide to try an unproven remedy, how should I proceed?

Before you decide to try an unproven remedy you should:
- Check with your doctor or local Arthritis Foundation chapter to find out what is known about the effects and safety of the remedy.
- Let your doctor know what you are thinking about trying. Don't be embarrassed. Your doctor knows your medical history and can help you look carefully at how safe a remedy may be for you. Continue your regular medical care for arthritis after careful discussion with your doctor.
- Remember that you play the most important role in your own care. You

make your own health-care decisions every day. As a consumer of health care, ask questions. Judge for yourself the effects and safety of any new treatment before you try it. You can ask your doctor or the Arthritis Foundation for more information on any treatment for arthritis.

• Agencies like the Arthritis Foundation, the Federal Drug Administration (FDA), and the Federal Trade Commission (FTC) can answer your questions or take your complaints about promoters of unproven remedies for arthritis. Your report of a problem may help keep an unsafe remedy off the market.

13

Arthritis Research

Progress in some areas of arthritis research is occurring so fast that the media often report new findings before medical journals containing the information can reach your doctor's office. As a result, you need to know how to evaluate reports on new arthritis research.

Arthritis researchers are looking at three broad areas of research: causes, treatments, and prevention. For example, researchers are trying to determine the causes of the early destruction of cartilage in osteoarthritis patients and ways to rebuild it. They are also trying to understand the steps that lead to inflammation in patients with diseases like rheumatoid arthritis and how it can be slowed or stopped.

Your doctor can tell you about new research findings. If you would like to take part in arthritis research, ask your doctor for a referral to a study in your area.

What agencies or companies are responsible for arthritis research?

Many people help make arthritis research possible. The federal government, through its National Institutes of Health (NIH) in Bethesda, Maryland, is the largest supporter of arthritis research. Drug companies do research on new medications.

The Arthritis Foundation is the largest private, nonprofit source of funds for arthritis research. Your contributions help the Arthritis Foundation support research and provide grants to train scientists and fund studies by experienced researchers. In addition, the Arthritis Foundation advocates strongly for government-sponsored arthritis research.

What major advances have been made in arthritis research in the last decade?

The improvement in the treatment of patients with rheumatoid arthritis through the use of methotrexate has been a major advance. Methotrexate was originally developed to treat leukemia and lymphoma, and high doses of methotrexate interfere with cancer cell growth. However, at lower doses (which greatly reduce the risk of serious side effects), methotrexate has been found to control RA symptoms and to limit the progression of disease. Over a 10-year period, researchers established that methotrexate is a safe and effective long-term treatment for RA.

Methotrexate slows the progression of joint deterioration, particularly if used early in the course of RA. In most cases it helps control the disease, and in some it may induce remission.

WHAT TO LOOK FOR IN NEWS ABOUT ARTHRITIS RESEARCH

WHEN YOU READ ABOUT A NEW FINDING IN ARTHRITIS RESEARCH, ASK THESE QUESTIONS:

- Is this research associated with a medical facility?

- Is there a scientific reason to think the results are reliable?

- Were the people in the study like you— the same age, sex and type of arthritis?

- Has the research been published in a medical journal?

- Does the report suggest health actions that people with your type of arthritis should take as a result of the research?

Have there been other changes recently in the treatment of rheumatoid arthritis?

For years, physicians withheld more potent drugs in the treatment of RA until after the patient had tried NSAIDs for a least a year or two. This approach was based on knowledge available at the time. New treatment options and new understanding of the disease process in RA has led physicians to revise the way they treat RA patients. It has been shown that joint damage in RA begins in the first seven years, so it's important to control the joint inflammation as early as possible.

The original treatment plan was often illustrated as a pyramid, with a base of NSAIDs, exercise, and rest. The next step was the disease-modifying anti-rheumatic drugs (DMARDs), including gold and antimalarials. If these were ineffective, more potent medications, such as methotrexate and penicillamine, were prescribed. At the top of the pyramid were experimental treatments and therapies. This path of treatment is no longer being pursued. Research has shown that NSAIDs do not halt the progression of RA, whereas drugs such as methotrexate and DMARDs can stop disease activity and progression. Now these drugs are being used earlier in the course of the illness. It is important that the diagnosis of RA be made early so that effective treatment can be used before joint damage has occurred.

What is the latest information on lupus research?

In the mid-1980s, researchers gave people with a form of lupus called lupus nephritis new hope with cyclophosphamide (*Cytoxan*) or CY, a chemical cousin to toxic mustard gas, combined with Prednisone.

In the 1960s, CY had been developed as an anti-cancer drug. Researchers noted that in addition to killing cancer cells, it suppressed the immune system. Because lupus is the result of an overactive immune system that turns against kidneys, skin, and joints, the question arose whether CY would help treat lupus.

Jack Klippel, MD, of the National Institutes of Health (NIH) in Bethesda, Maryland, and his colleagues at NIH have studied the effect of CY, given both orally and intravenous in monthly doses, on the inflamed kidneys of patients with lupus. In 1986, they reported in the *New England Journal of Medicine* that CY plus Prednisone controlled kidney damage in nearly three-fourths of the patients to whom this combination was given. These results have been confirmed.

CY has serious side effects, however, such as sterility, cancer, and increased risk of infection. Consequently, its use must be weighed carefully and monitored appropriately. Researchers hope these side effects can be reduced through intravenous administration.

What's new in research on the connection between genetics and arthritis?

Research has established that genetics play a role in the development of RA, as well as in the development of ankylosing spondylitis. The genetic marker HLA-B27 is associated with ankylosing spondylitis, and genetic marker HLA-DR4 is linked with RA. Still, having either marker does not guarantee that disease will develop.

According to Cornelia Weyand, MD, PhD, of the Mayo Clinic, HLA-DR4 is only one marker for RA. Isolating a series of markers could help physicians learn more about the course of the disease in a patient. Understanding the other genes involved in RA is the next step in research. Once that information is known, it may be possible for physicians to predict which patients are likely to have more severe disease.

Other important work in genetics has focused on studies of twins, which usually serve as the "gold standard" for determining whether a disease is genetic in nature. Theoretically, any genetic disease that occurs in one identical twin should occur in both, but it hasn't worked out this way with RA patients. Researchers have argued that twins must have differing environmental exposures to infectious agents. A susceptibility for the disease is inherited. But something else, a virus or a bacterial infection, sets the illness in motion.

Unlike RA, where multiple genes and other factors may be involved, in patients with some of the rare types of osteoarthritis that have a genetic basis, a genetic abnormality (a mutation or change in the gene) exists and everyone who has the abnormality gets the disease.

In 1990, Roland Moskowitz, MD professor of medicine at Case Western Reserve University in Cleveland, and Darwin J. Prockop, MD of Jefferson Medical College in Philadelphia, discovered that a mutation in the collagen II gene caused the involved person to produce defective cartilage that was prone to breakdown. As a result, people carrying the faulty collagen gene develop osteoarthritis in their twenties and often have to have joint replacements by their forties. Since that discovery, researchers have found inherited OA in a number of families with different mutations in the collagen II gene and in associated genes.

What's new in osteoporosis research?

Researchers have learned over the last decade that people who attain the highest bone density by the age of 35 have the lowest risk of developing osteoporosis. Heredity plays a role in a person's maximum bone density, and we have no control over that fact. Estrogen is a key factor in slowing bone loss, and consequently women in the menopausal period are at high risk for developing osteoporosis. It has been shown that the use of estrogen in the postmenopausal period reduces bone loss and the resulting fractures. In addition, studies have shown that taking certain actions, such as improving your calcium intake, getting enough vitamin D, exercising, and refraining from smoking, can help increase overall bone density.

Before the development of the various bone scans to detect early osteoporosis, physicians could detect the disease only after a patient had sustained a fracture. There was no way of determining who was at risk of developing the disease. Now bone scans, such as the dual-energy X-ray absorptiometry (the DEXA imaging method), can detect loss of bone density, which indicates whether a person is at risk of developing fractures from osteoporosis.

In 1995, a new drug, alendronate *(Fosamax)*, was introduced for the prevention of osteoporosis. This drug slows the demineralization or breakdown of bone. Another drug introduced for use in people with osteoporosis is intranasal calcitonin, which also slows bone breakdown. While alendronate and calcitonin offer significant advances in treating osteoporosis, they don't build new, healthy bone. In the future new drugs may be developed that will actually build new bone.

Is it true that some joint damage can be repaired with replacement cartilage?

A widely publicized therapy for OA involves taking healthy cartilage cells from a knee, placing those cells in a special culture solution where they reproduce to about 10 times their original number, and then implanting the newly grown cells in the damaged area. The procedure, which was developed in Sweden, is now being performed at about 10 U.S. medical centers. It's used primarily to repair small cartilage defects caused by injury. The long-term benefits of this procedure are not yet known.

Other researchers have focused on the molecular mechanisms that are associated with the breakdown of cartilage. Such studies may eventually allow doctors to make an early diagnosis of cartilage damage. By understanding the mechanism of cartilage breakdown, drugs may be designed to interrupt this breakdown and turn off the destructive process.

I've heard that agents called biologic disease modifiers are being used experimentally to treat people with RA. What is the status of this?

New drugs show promise in blocking the biological processes that perpetuate the joint inflammation and destruction in rheumatoid arthritis. These drugs are known as biologic response modifiers, and some are genetically-engineered agents that interfere with the inflammatory process in rheumatoid arthritis.

One such agent is tumor necrosis factor (TNF) receptor, a biologic response modifier currently being studied in RA patients. TNF is a protein that is a key messenger in the body's chemical chain reaction that leads to inflammation. By blocking the production of TNF or inhibiting its activity, it is possible to stop the inflammatory process.

Another biologic response modifier is recombinant human Interleukin-1 receptor antagonist (IL-1). IL-1 is another key substance involved in the inflammatory chain reaction in rheumatoid arthritis. Blocking the activity of IL-1 may reduce or halt the inflammation and destruction of a joint affected by RA.

Is there any research that shows what impact physical activity can have on patients with fibromyalgia?

People with fibromyalgia who cut back on their activity become deconditioned. This can lead to pain and an increase in fatigue, which can lead to even more reduced physical activity.

Researchers from Oregon Health Services University in Portland concluded that exercise could actually ease the pain and fatigue of fibromyalgia and improve the likelihood that patients would be able to maintain their regular levels of activity. Several more studies have been conducted, all of which came to the same conclusion.

What has research found out about the link between weight loss and osteoarthritis?

In the last few years, researchers from Boston University Arthritis Center reported some of their findings from what is known as the Framingham Study. By studying the health histories of a large number of people, they confirmed that excess weight can induce or aggravate arthritis. In addition, they found that losing weight before symptoms occur can actually reduce the risk of developing osteoarthritis of the knee. This was the first time that a specific lifestyle change had been linked to the prevention of a major type of arthritis.

14

Working with Arthritis: Your Legal Rights

Federal laws have made the playing field more level for people with arthritis and other disabling conditions who wish to remain employed. The Americans with Disabilities Act of 1990 and its predecessor, the Rehabilitation Act of 1973, give important protections to workers in the private sector and the federal government.

The new Family and Medical Leave Act also provides relief to workers faced with lengthy absences because of illness. Your state may have additional laws that further protect people with disabilities from discrimination.

If you are having difficulty on your job because of arthritis or another rheumatic disease, this chapter will help you understand your legal rights, suggest ways to gain support from your employer and co-workers, and give you ideas for ways to make your work easier.

What legal rights do I have?

The Americans with Disabilities Act (ADA), passed by the U.S. Congress in 1990, is the most extensive bill of rights for people with disabilities ever signed into law. It bans discrimination against people with disabilities in many areas, including hiring and employment.

At the same time, it protects employers from having to make changes that are unreasonable or expensive. These changes are called unreasonable accommodations.

What are reasonable or unreasonable accommodations?

Reasonable accommodations are changes that are needed to enable you to apply for a job, perform the essential functions of the job, and enjoy the benefits and privileges of employment. Examples of reasonable accommodations include allowing you to shift to a part-time or adjusted work schedule; restructuring your job; providing you with an accessible parking space; providing assistive equipment/devices; providing greater access to the work site (such as an access ramp); and/or making changes in the height of your desk. If you have arthritis, any or all of these reasonable accommodations should be at your disposal to enable you to perform your job.

Changes that would put undue hardship (defined as significant difficulty or expense) on an employer are considered unreasonable accommodations. If the cost of making the accommodation is an undue hardship for the employer, he or she must give you the choice of providing it for yourself or sharing in the cost. The employer cannot ask you to pay for reasonable accommodations, and he or she cannot pay you less to cover their cost.

Keep in mind that an employer is not required to place you in a particular job if he or she believes that doing so would put you or others at increased risk.

What types of companies does the ADA apply to?

The ADA applies to companies that employ fifteen or more people. It bans discrimination against qualified individuals with disabilities by private employers, state and local governments, employment agencies, and labor unions. It applies to all aspects of employment, including hiring, job assignments, training, promotion, pay, benefits, and company-sponsored social events.

What qualifications have to be met to be considered disabled?

For you to be considered an individual with a disability, arthritis must "substantially limit" a major life activity, such as walking, performing manual tasks, or working. To be considered qualified for a specific position, you must still have the education, skill, and experience the employer requires. You must also be able to perform the essential functions of the job that are listed in an advertised job description, with or without reasonable accommodation.

How can I make the ADA work for me?

The ADA and the legal rights it creates give you the tools to be an effective advocate for yourself. You should be able to work with your employer for your mutual benefit.

If you feel that you haven't been treated fairly, the ADA allows you to file complaints with the Equal Employment Opportunity Commission (EEOC) and other federal agencies. However, the ADA also encourages other ways of settling disagreements, such as negotiation, mediation, mini-trials, and arbitration. Considering these alternative approaches makes good sense since litigation may be time-consuming and costly, and you still may not achieve your goal.

What is the Rehabilitation Act of 1973 and how does it help me?

The Rehabilitation Act of 1973 was the model for the ADA, and it contains many of the same protections for people with disabilities. It applies to the federal government and all its agencies, to companies that do business with the government, and to institutions that receive federal financial assistance.

What is the Family and Medical Leave Act?

The Family and Medical Leave Act (FMLA), which went into effect in August 1993, includes a provision that allows employees to take up to three months of unpaid medical leave per year if they are unable to work because of a serious health condition. You can take FMLA leave all at one time, at different periods, or by working part-time.

The FMLA applies to companies that employ 50 or more workers within a 75-mile radius.

To be eligible for family leave, you must have worked for your employer for 1,250 hours in the previous 12 months. Whenever possible, you should provide advance leave notice and medical certification.

How can the FMLA help me?

Your employer must allow you to take unpaid leave to care for a newborn, an adopted, or a foster child; to care for a spouse, child, or parent who has a serious health condition; or to care for your own serious health condition.

You may take intermittent leave or work a reduced leave schedule (fewer hours per day) with employer approval. When you return to work, in most cases you must be restored to your original or equivalent position, with equivalent pay, benefits, and other terms of employment. Your medical insurance benefits must be continued on the same terms.

It is against the law for your employer to interfere with or deny rights granted under the FMLA. All employers are required to post notices of rights under the FMLA.

What is vocational rehabilitation?

The goal of vocational rehabilitation is to help people with disabilities develop job skills and find and keep employment. It has been found to have a 50 percent success rate in helping people with arthritis find employment.

VR services vary from state to state but usually include counseling and guidance about possible careers, transportation assistance, help in obtaining assistive devices (such as wheelchairs), and assistance in learning how to use tools, equipment, and supplies and in obtaining licenses you need to perform your work. VR services also usually include job training, job placement, and personal assistance services.

What are the possibilities of working from home?

If you are independent and self-disciplined and like to plan your own hours, a home business may be right for you. You might telecommute for an employer or start your own business.

If you feel confident that you can handle your own small business, contact the Small Business Administration office (SBA) in your area. The SBA's Handicapped Assistance Loan (HAL-2) program provides direct loans and loan guarantees to qualified individuals with disabilities to set up their own businesses. The agency also provides individual guidance and a variety of classes for people starting their own businesses. Many college and community adult education programs offer similar classes.

I really enjoy my present job. What are some suggestions for managing my arthritis at work?

Combined with getting good medical care, you should be flexible, creative, and a problem solver who can help balance work and the demands of arthritis. This is, of course, an ongoing and possibly evolving process. Start by figuring out your energy patterns during the day and what kinds of activities hurt or help you. Discuss this with your employer and get suggestions about time management and changes that might be necessary in the work place. The following suggestions might also be helpful:

- Create an efficient work environment by arranging things around you to limit the amount of lifting, reaching, carrying, walking, and holding you must do.
- Set priorities and pace yourself by listing the tasks that you must do, in order of their importance. Do the important tasks when you feel strongest and most energetic.
- Vary your activities from time to time so that you do not sit for too long in a single position.
- Keep a diary of good and bad days to help predict the causes that may tend to trigger flares.
- Maintain a positive attitude by focusing on your abilities. Keeping a sense of humor and paying attention to your appearance can also boost your self-esteem and help you keep a professional image.
- By all means try to maintain a schedule that helps you avoid fatigue at work. Get plenty of rest to carry you through the day. Include exercise, therapy, and regular medical check-ups in your schedule.

Can my computer be made arthritis-friendly?

Yes, the computer can be made arthritis-friendly if you adjust the way you use it. Taking short breaks from your work from time to time can help prevent problems. Stretching your arm and finger muscles before you begin working and during breaks can also help. Computers have made life at work easier, but those who use them for long periods of time may feel stress on joints and tendons in the arms, wrists, and fingers. Proper seating, assistive devices, and clever use of all the labor-saving shortcuts your computer offers can also help limit stress on your joints and increase your productivity.

Can special devices really help manage arthritis at work?

Special devices really can help. Keep in mind that "reasonable accommo-dations" under the ADA are defined as those that will not cause undue hardship on your employer, meaning that they are not too difficult or too expensive to provide. Costs of equipment vary, but some equipment will probably fall into the category of reasonable accommodations that will help you do and keep your job. In fact, you may be able to get funding for the devices you need through your insurance company, federal or state agencies (such as Medicare), or vocational rehabilitation or service organizations.

Resources

About the Arthritis Foundation

The Arthritis Foundation is the source of help and hope for nearly 40 million Americans who have arthritis. Founded in 1948, the Arthritis Foundation is the only national, voluntary health organization that works for all people affected by any of the more than 100 forms of arthritis or related diseases. Volunteers in chapters nationwide help to support research, professional and community education programs, services for people with arthritis, government advocacy and fund-raising activities.

The American Juvenile Arthritis Organization (AJAO) is composed of children, parents, teachers and others concerned specifically with juvenile arthritis. A council of the Arthritis Foundation, AJAO focuses its efforts on the problems related to arthritis in children.

The focus of the Arthritis Foundation is twofold: to support research to find the cure for and prevention of arthritis, and to improve the quality of life for those affected by arthritis. Public contributions enable the Arthritis Foundation to fulfill this mission — in fact, at least 80 cents of every dollar donated to the Arthritis Foundation serves to directly fund research and program services.

The Arthritis Foundation Helps

Arthritis doesn't have to rob you of the activities you enjoy most. While research holds the key to future cures or preventions for arthritis, equally important is improving the quality of life for people with arthritis today. Your local Arthritis Foundation has information, classes and other services to put you in charge of your arthritis. The Arthritis Foundation has more than 150 local offices across the United States. To find an office near you, and to determine which of the following resources are available through your nearest chapter, call 800/283-7800.

Medical and Self-Care Programs

1. Physician referral - Most Arthritis Foundation chapters can give you a list of doctors in your area who specialize in the evaluation and treatment of arthritis and arthritis-related diseases.
2. Exercise programs - Recreational in nature, these are developed, coordinated and sponsored by the Arthritis Foundation. All have specially trained instructors. Programs include:

• Joint Efforts - This arthritis movement program teaches gentle, undemanding movement exercises for people with arthritis, including those who use walkers and wheelchairs. Joint Efforts is designed to encourage movement and socialization among older adults and to help decrease pain, stiffness and depression.

• PACE (People with Arthritis Can Exercise) - PACE is an exercise program that uses gentle activities to help increase joint flexibility, range of motion and stamina, and to help maintain muscle strength. Two videotapes showing basic and advanced levels of the program are available from your local chapter for preview or for practice at home. To purchase the videos, call 800/933-0032; $15.75 and $4.00 shipping and handling for members; $19.50 and $4.00 shipping and handling for non-members.

• Arthritis Foundation Aquatic Program - Originally co-developed by the YMCA and the Arthritis Foundation, this water exercise program helps relieve the strain on muscles and joints for people with arthritis. The PEP (Pool Exercise Program) video-tape shows how to exercise on your own. To order the video, call 800/933-0032; $15.75 and $4.00 shipping and handling for members; $19.50 and $4.00 shipping and handling for non-members.

Educational and Support Groups

1. Arthritis Foundation Support and Education Groups - These are mutual-support groups that provide opportunities for discussion and problem solving. They are usually formed by people with arthritis and/or their family members who wish to meet with their peers for mutual assistance in satisfying common needs and in overcoming problems related to arthritis.

2. Classes/courses - Formal group meetings help people with various forms of arthritis gain the knowledge, skills and confidence they need to actively manage their conditions. Courses focus on proper exercises, medications, relaxation techniques, pain management, dealing with depression, nutrition, nontraditional treatments and doctor-patient relations. The classes include:

- Arthritis Self-Help Course
- Fibromyalgia Self-Help Course
- Systemic Lupus Erythematosus Self-Help Course

Reliable Information At Your Fingertips

1. Information hotline - The Arthritis Foundation is *the* expert on arthritis and is only a phone call away. Call toll free at 800/283-7800 for automated information on arthritis 24 hours a day. Trained volunteers and staff are also available at your local Arthritis Foundation chapter to answer your questions or send you a list of physicians in your area who specialize in arthritis.

2. Arthritis Foundation Web Site - Information about arthritis is available 24 hours a day to Internet users via the Arthritis Foundation's site on the World Wide Web. The address for the web site is http://www.arthritis.org.

address for the web site is http://www.arthritis.org.

3. Publications - A number of publications are available to educate people with arthritis and their families and friends about important considerations such as medications, exercise, diet, pain management and stress management, to name a few.

• Books - Self-help books by the Arthritis Foundation are available to help you learn more about your condition and how to manage it. Check your local bookstores, your local Arthritis Foundation chapter, or order a book through the Arthritis Foundation by calling 800/207-8633.

• Booklets - More than 60 booklets and brochures provide information on the many arthritis-related diseases and conditions, medications, how to work with your doctor, and how to care for yourself. Single copies are available free of charge. Call 800/283-7800 for a free listing of booklets on arthritis.

• *Arthritis Today* - The award-winning bimonthly magazine *Arthritis Today* gives you the latest information on research, new treatments and tips from experts and readers to help you manage arthritis. Each issue also brings you a variety of helpful and interesting articles covering diet and nutrition, tips for traveling, and ways you can make your life with arthritis easier and more rewarding. A one-year subscription to *Arthritis Today* is yours free when you become a member of the Arthritis Foundation. You'll also have access to a wide range of local chapter activities. Annual membership is $20 and helps fund research to find cures for arthritis. Call 800/933-0032 for membership and subscription information.

4. Audiovisual libraries - Available either on loan or for purchase, a number of audio- and video-cassettes cover a variety of topics from exercise to relaxation. Call your local chapter for a listing of titles, prices and availabilities.

5. Public forums - Educational programs are presented to the community on various requested topics.

6. Professional publications - A number of professional education materials on arthritis geared to the health-care professional are available through the Arthritis Foundation. These materials, including the 356-page *Primer on the Rheumatic Diseases*, which is published every five years, are available by calling 800/207-8633.

Remember the Arthritis Foundation in your will.

The mission of the Arthritis Foundation is to support arthritis research and to improve the quality of life for those affected by it. Planned giving is an important part of this mission. The Foundation's planned giving department offers a wide variety of gift planning options, including estate gifts and gifts that provide donors with lifetime income. We hope that you decide to include a gift to the Foundation in your will. For more information, call the Arthritis Foundation's planned giving department at 404/872-7100.

Arthritis Foundation
1330 West Peachtree Street
Atlanta, GA 30309
404-872-7100
http://www.arthritis.org

NOTES

NOTES